EYELASH EXTENSIONS
TRAINING FROM THE BEST

BEGINNER'S TRAINING MANUAL

JESSICA COX

Copyright 2016
Seattle, Wa

All rights reserved. No part of this publication may be reproduced, distributed or trasmitted in any form or by any means, including photocopying, recording or other electronic or mechanical methods, without prior written permission of Fringe Beneyefits. Exception: brief quotations embodied in articles and certain other non commercial uses permitted by copyright law.

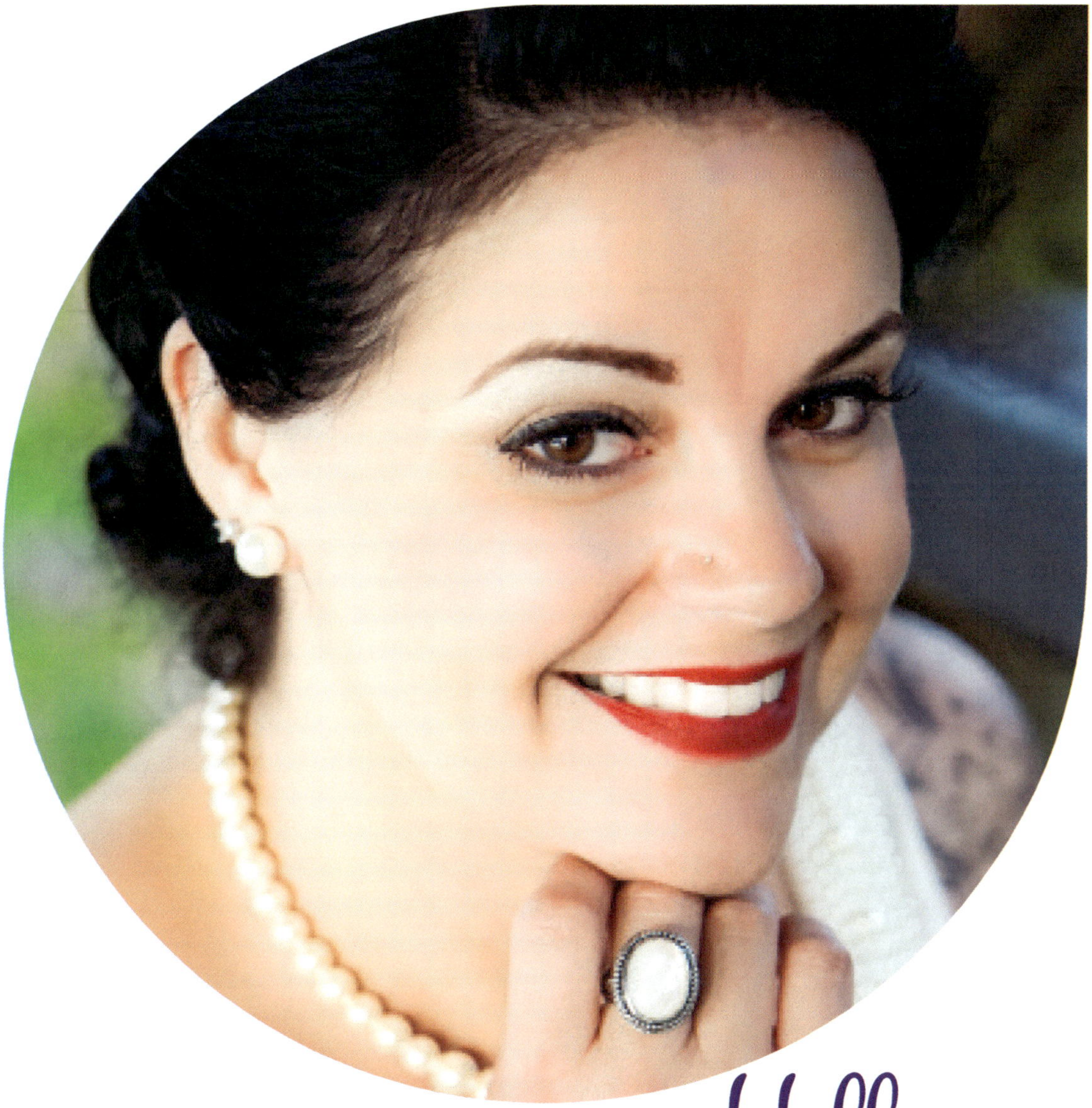

Hello

Meet Jessie

My name is Jessie Cox. I have been a beauty professional for over a decade and have been creating beautiful eyes with eyelash extensions since 2007. I've trained with top experts in the field and have certifications from three different organizations.

This program was created after seeing a need for comprehensive training for beginners and experts alike. You can't be too careful with people's eyes.

Your Future is Beautiful

Congratulations on your decision to further your skills, knowledge and earning potential by becoming an eyelash extensions expert with Fringe Beneyefits. It is my goal to give you the best possible training. I have seen the eyelash extension industry explode and the training from one company to the next varies... considerably! Good Training = Beautiful Lashes

So together we will cover the basics to make sure you know everything you need to about eyelash extensions. This will be a considerable amount of information because I have found without a solid knowledge of how eyelash extensions work, people don't have what they need to build proper skills.

We will cover everything there is to know about eyelash extension materials and sizing. Next we will go over eyelash extension adhesives and specifically our five Glues. Also Primers, De-Fringe Adhesive Remover and our newest addition Lash Ready Extension Bond Enhancer. Consent forms and proper set-up will round out the training until we get to application. You will be given instructions on the correct procedures for applying eyelash extensions individually so you can begin to practice and develop your skills correctly.
We will cover full sets and fills.

The training will be wrapped up with commonly seen problems and the do's and don'ts of eyelash extensions. Advanced training covering colored lashes, glitter/gems and the advanced techniques of picking different looks for your clients will be offered in another class after you get the basics down.

Mink training is also available. Our True Sable Siberian mink fur and fox fur, gently harvested of course, not faux mink. Faux mink is synthetic premium silk. At Fringe Beneyefits premium is our standard.

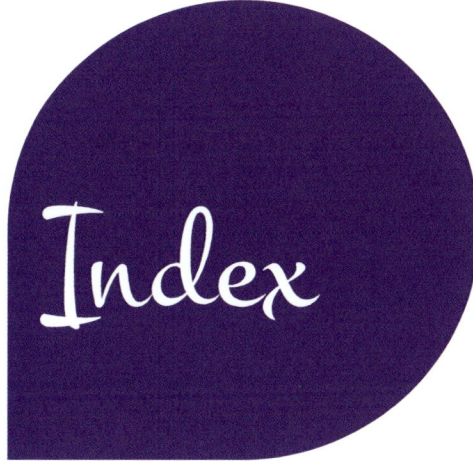

Index

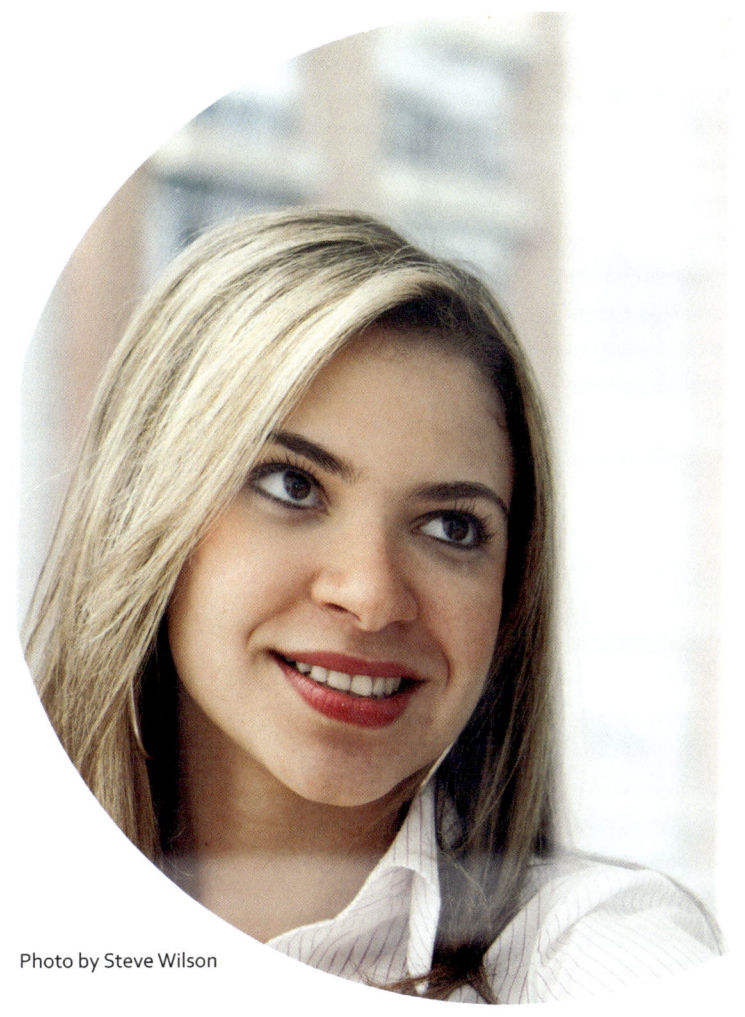

Photo by Steve Wilson

- The Basics
- Lashes
- Glues (Adhesives)
- Consultation
- Application

The Basics

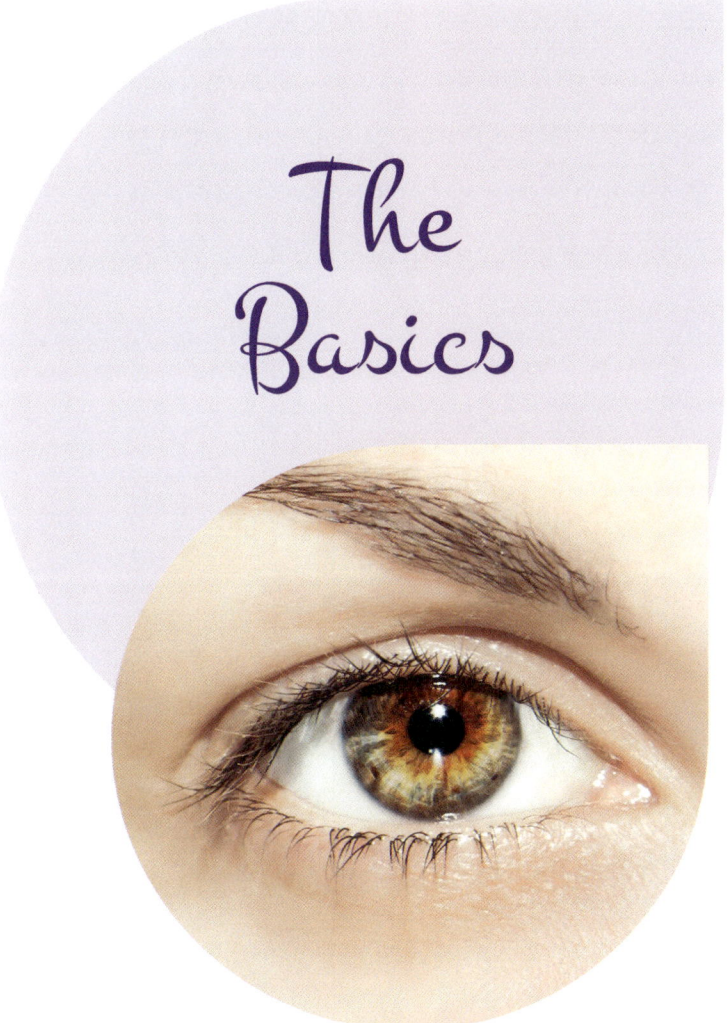
Before

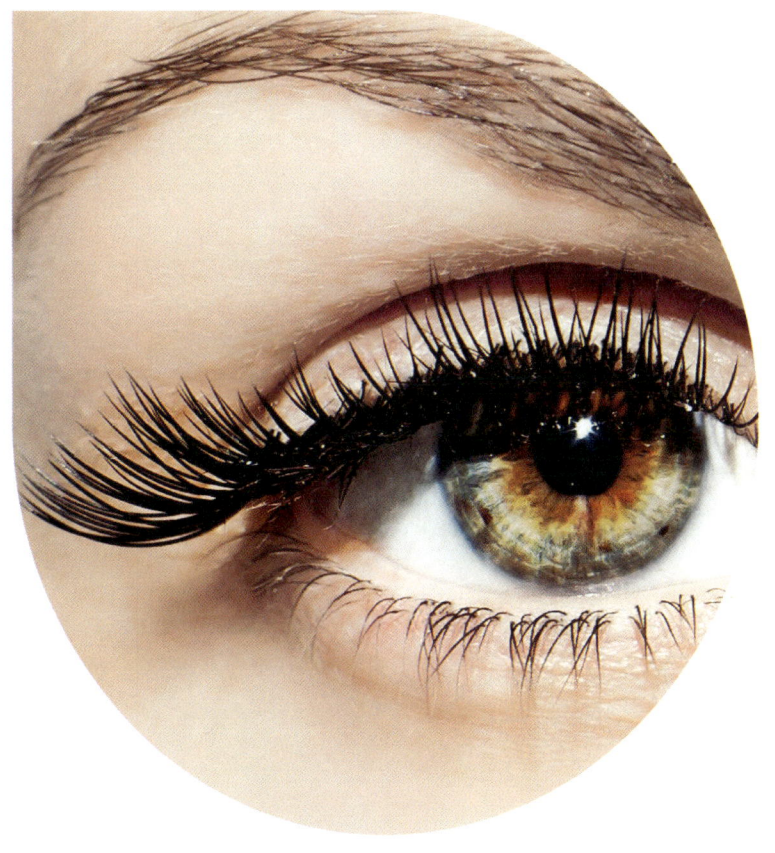
After

What are eyelash extensions?

Lash Extensions are hair-by-hair extensions of your natural eye lashes.

Eyelash Extensions are a great way to extend the length and thickness of your eyelashes. They are applied on a hair-by-hair one-to-one basis to your own eyelashes for a very natural look. It is a very precise service that requires great skill, with the use of the highest quality products. At Fringe Beneyefits our extensions are the softest synthetic lashes available, made from silk. These are not strips or cluster eyelashes. Eyelash extensions are never applied to the skin. Once applied, correctly, these eyelash extensions are so natural looking it is difficult to tell, even up close, that you have extensions on.

We are also now proud to offer True Sable 100% Siberian mink fur eyelash extensions that are gently harvested and cruelty free.

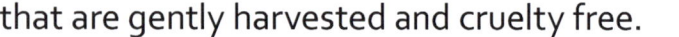

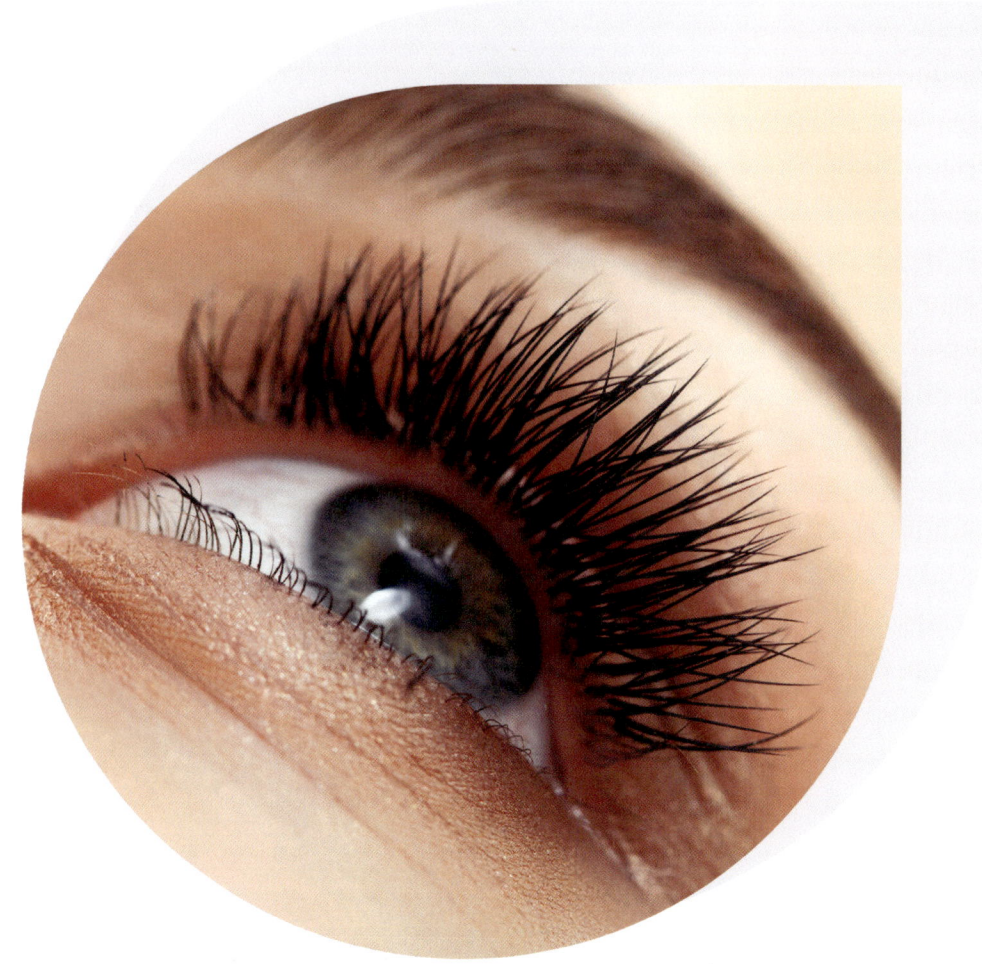

Who Are They For? Anyone!

Lash extensions can be as different as each client. The possibilities are endless.

Busy Women

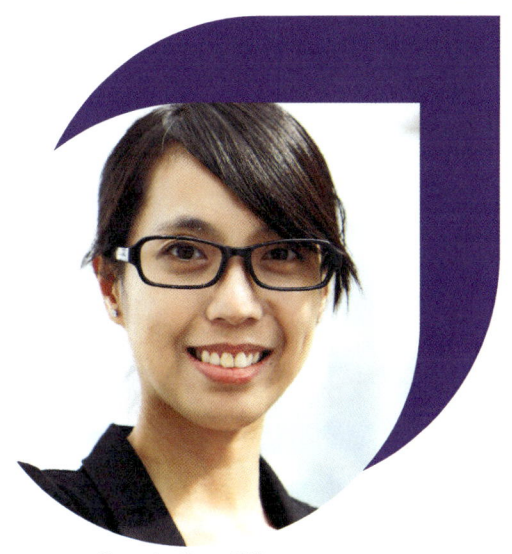

Photo by Steve Wilson

Athletes

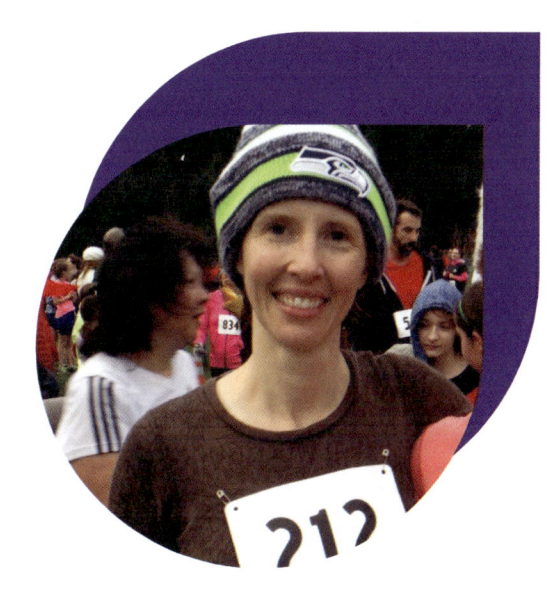

Brides

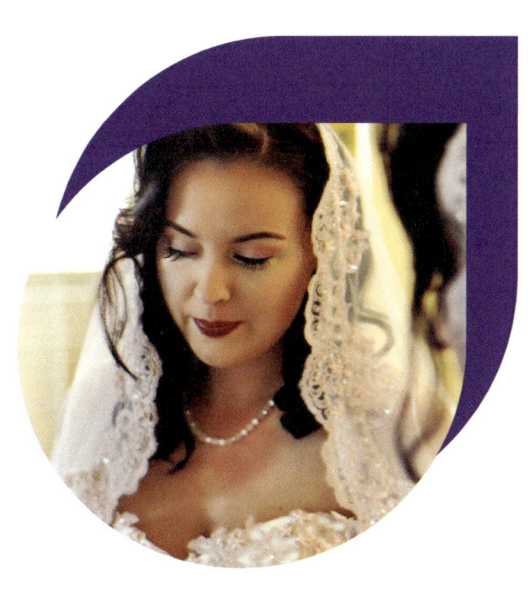

Anyone!

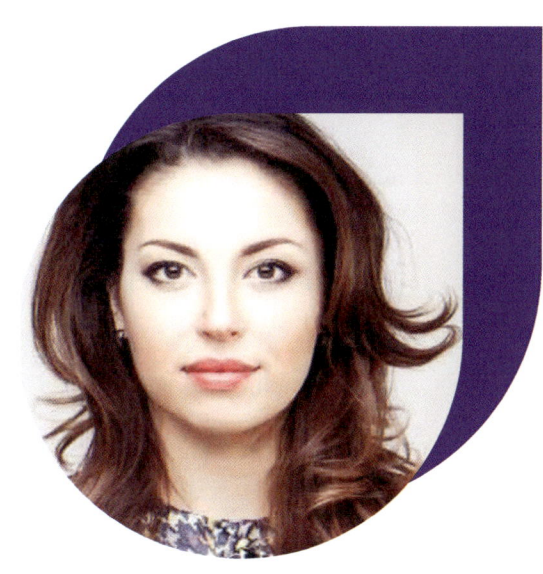

Why Does Everyone Want Them?

"I don't like Mascara. It's messy."

"My makeup just sweats off at practice."

"I don't want to worry about makeup on my vacation."

"I want to look perfect for my wedding day!"

"At my age, I have started thinking about anti-aging"

"Who wants to mess with mascara all the time?"

"I want to do something fun for the party this weekend."

"I'm always in the water. Mascara just comes off."

"I don't have time for makeup in the mornings."

"I end up looking like a racoon by lunchtime."

"I'm so clumsy I never get my makeup right."

"I'm not looking any younger."

"My eyelashes are invisible!"

"Just because I'm a boy, doesn't mean I can't look fabulous!"

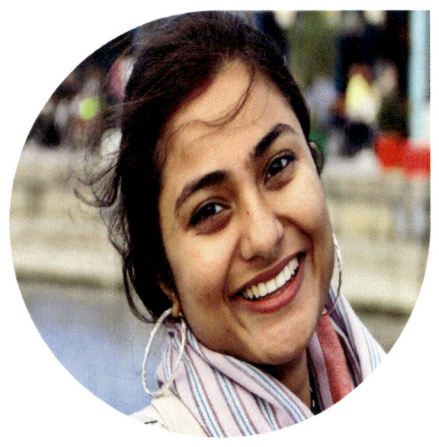
Photo by Debarski Ray

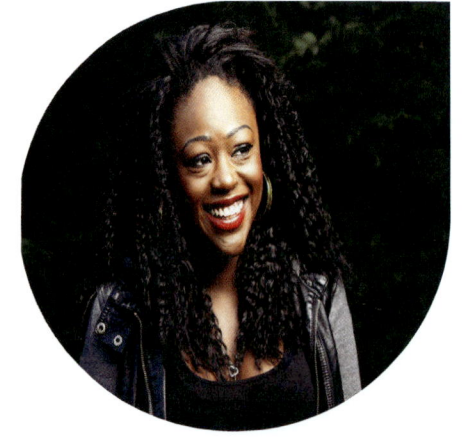
Photo by Sibok M. Patenaude

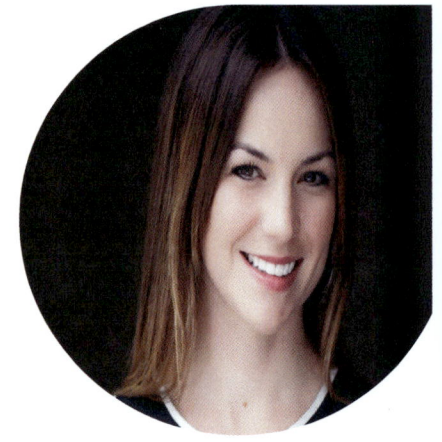
Photo by Nan Palmero

How do eyelash extensions work?

Eyelash extensions are glued to the individual eyelash, approximately 1mm away from the skin (a dime's width). Therefore when the natural eyelash falls out, the eyelash extension goes right along with it.

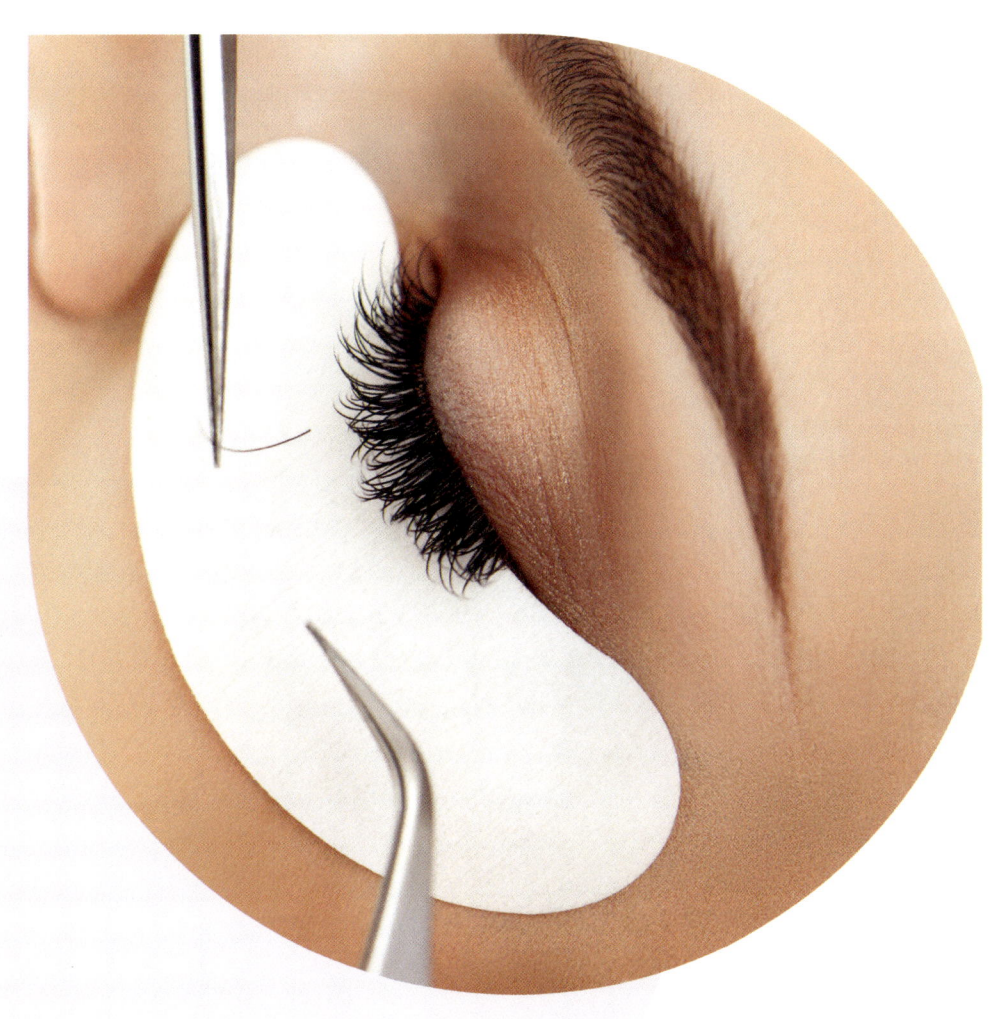

Key Facts

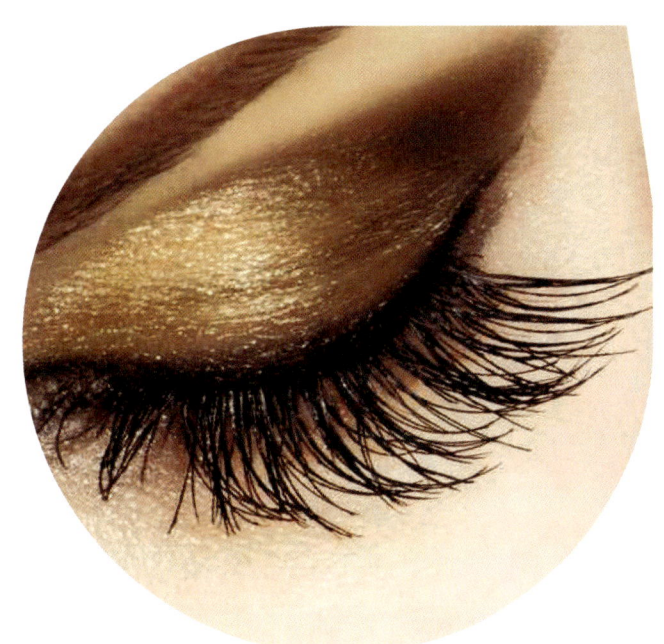

Extensions are replenished every 2-3 weeks.

After 2-3 weeks clients notice 1/3 to 1/2 of their extensions have shed. That is the time to come in and have a fill on all the newly grown in natural eyelashes.

Extensions are attached to each natural

A common misconception is that the extension is pulling the natural lash out. No! The client should see her own lash attached to the extension when it falls out because they fall out together. Now she will notice every little lash she loses because there is an extension

Eyelashes have a 6-8 week lifecycle.

Your natural eyelashes grow in, hang out and then fall off. Constantly. Of course everyone varies just a little bit. Hormones, vitamins and supplements can affect hair growth. If she is noticing a difference in the hair on her head or body hair, chances are her eyelashes are doing the same thing. An example of this can be about 3 months after childbirth most mothers notice a shedding. While she is losing the hair on her head, she may notice more eyelashes falling out as well.

Only put extensions on mature lashes.

You should not put synthetic eyelash extensions on eyelashes that are just starting to grow in. If they are significantly shorter than the other eyelashes, leave them alone. They will not be able to handle the weight of the extension. They will either fall off immediately or droop, hang or twist.

Essential Supplies

Fringe Beneyefits – Basic Starter Kit

6 Jars Premium Extensions:
- J-Curl .15 x 9mm
- J-Curl .15 x 11mm
- J-Curl .15 x 13mm
- J-Curl .15 x 15mm
- C-Curl .15 x 11mm
- C-Curl .15 x 13mm
- 2 x Straight Tweezers
- Curved Tweezers
- Sensitive Bond Glue
- Primer
- Lash Ready
- Lash Ready Wands
- De-Fringe Gel Remover
- Paper Tape Roll
- Plastic Tape Roll
- Crystal Pallet
- Silicone Mat
- Eyewash Pump
- 5 Gel Eyepads
- Mascara Wands

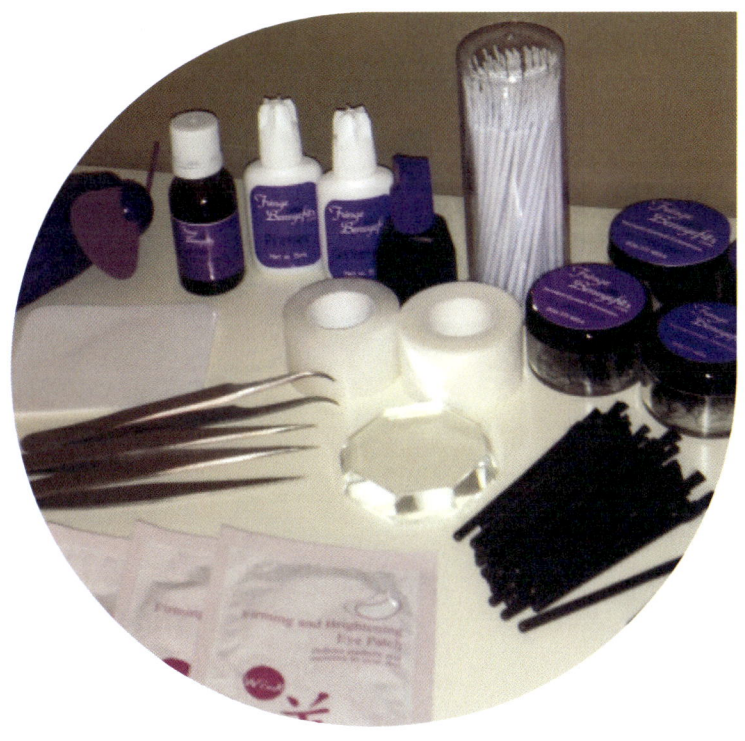

Fringe Beneyefits – Deluxe Add On Kit

- J-Curl .10 x 10mm, J-Curl .10 x 12mm,
- J-Curl .10 x 14mm, J-Curl .20 x 11mm,
- J-Curl .20 x 13mm, J-Curl .20 x 15mm,
- C-Curl .15 x 15mm, C-Curl .20 x 11mm,
- C-Curl .20 x 13mm, C-Curl .20 x 15mm,
- Eyelash Extension Sealant
- Sealant Brushes

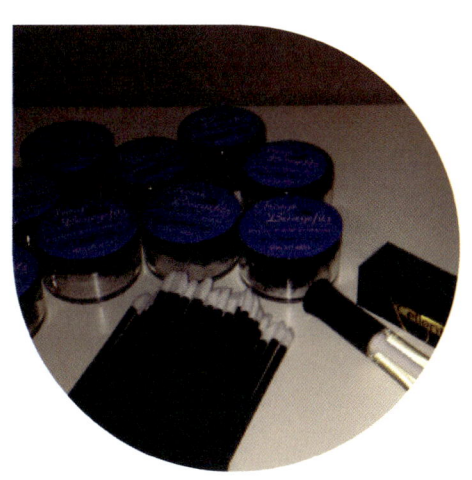

It's your job to decide...

who should get lashes.

- Healthy eyes
- Healthy eyelashes
- Healthy skin around the eyes
- Normal to oily skin-not too oily
- Realistic expectations

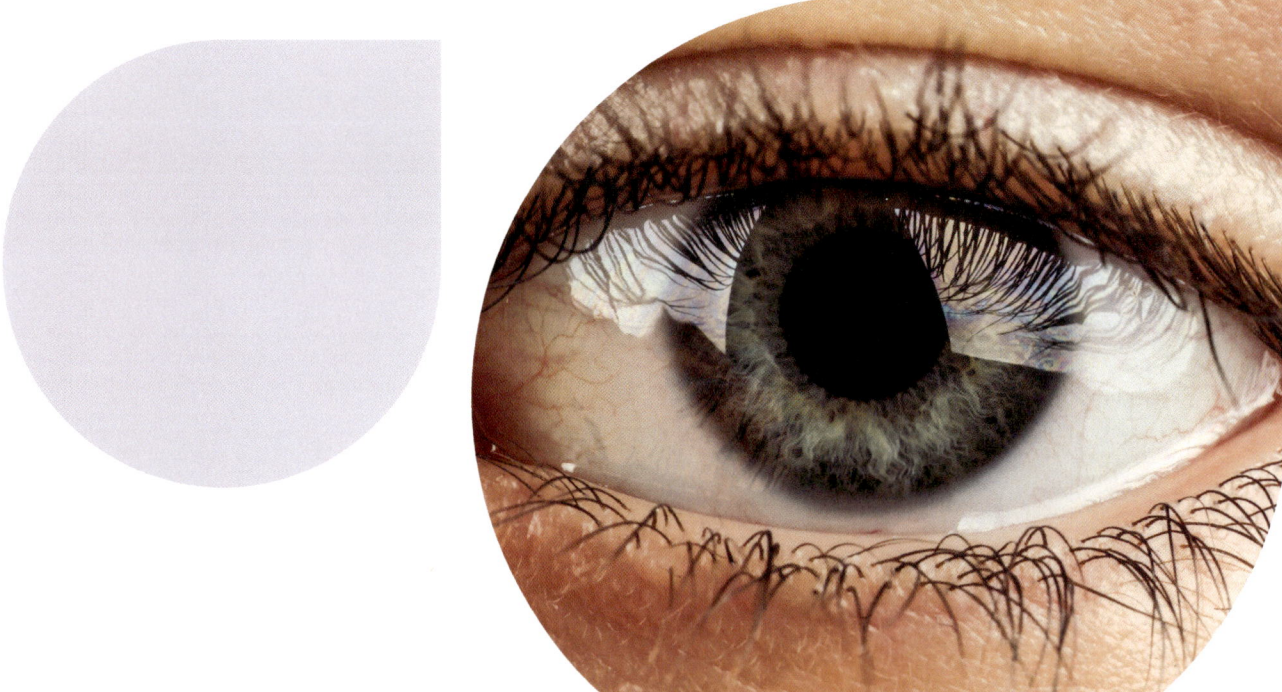

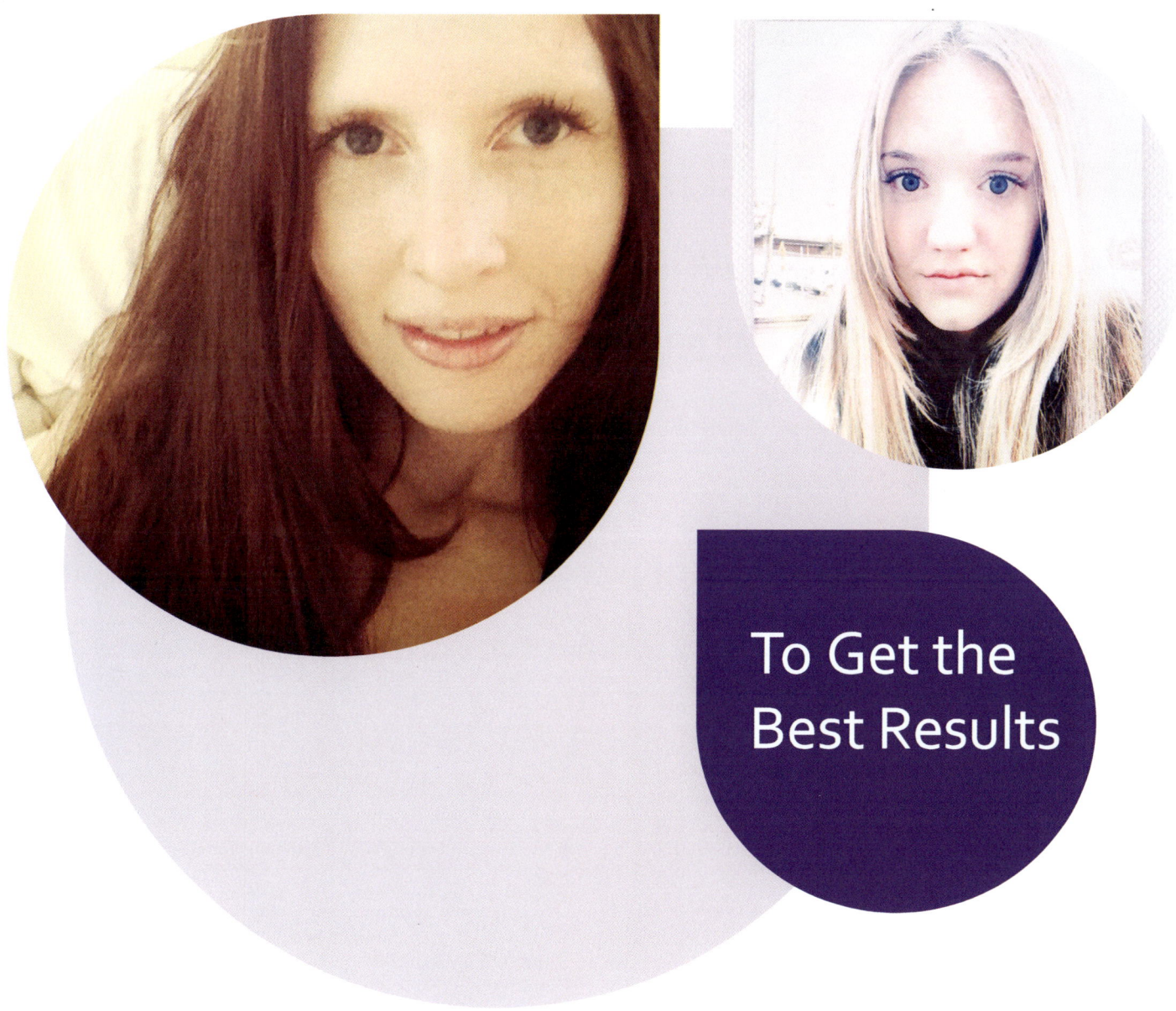

To Get the Best Results

Note: Some permanent cosmetics technicians ask that eyelash extensions be removed completely before the procedure. Some will work with the extensions. It's really up to the technician and what she is most comfortable with, there is no right way or wrong way. It may sometimes vary from client to client and what she is doing. For example if she really wants to get in the lash line she'll ask for removal, but if its just touching up a thick line, then the client can leave them on. Again, it's the personal preference of the permanent cosmetics technician. No one else should form an opinion- including us!!

It's your job to decide...
who should NOT.

- Unhealthy eyes
- Unhealthy eyelashes
- Thin or sensitive skin around the eyes*
- Want a heavy false lash look
- Can't follow directions

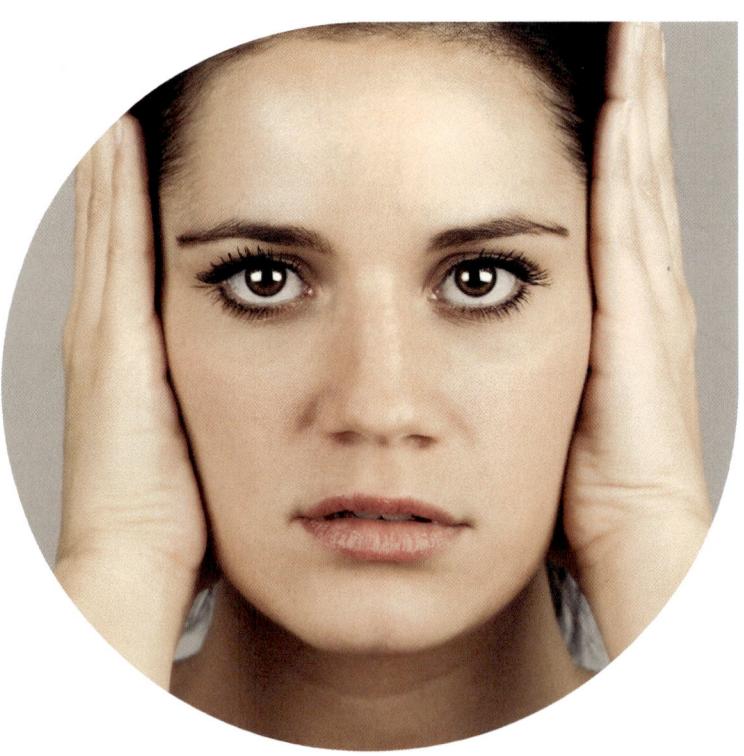

*Note: It's important to ask your clients if they have had or are receiving any of the following treatments: Recent LASIK surgery, eye-lift, chemical peel, Retin-A, Accutane, acne medications that thin the skin, and recent permanent cosmetics. Usually permanent cosmetics are healed after 5 days. If they have had or are using any of these treatments, they might not be a good canidate. Be gentle and respectful, but firm when declining a client. These are their eyes. "Betsy, I'm really sorry to tell you this. I don't think you are a good candidate for eyelash extensions because <reason>. I'd like you to talk to your doctor and have her clear you."

Make Case by Case Decisions

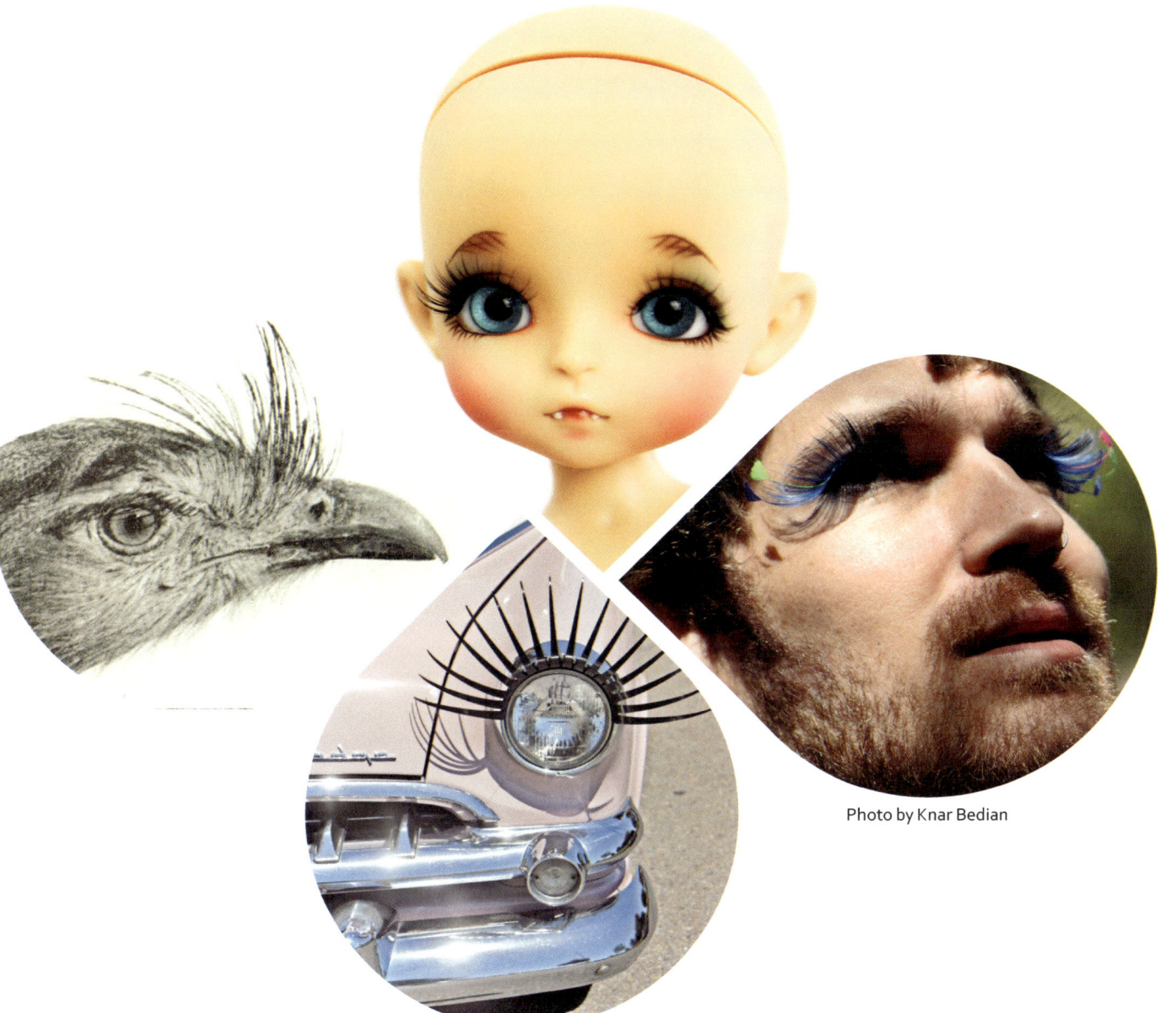

Photo by ThePeachPeddler

Photo by Knar Bedian

Photo by torbakhopper

Note: Some men do in fact wear eyelash extensions and we think that is fabulous. We refer to clients as she throughout the manual for ease but would never discriminate or withhold services based on gender. The lashes shown to the right are too long and obviously strip lashes, we would not be able to give him that look with extenions.

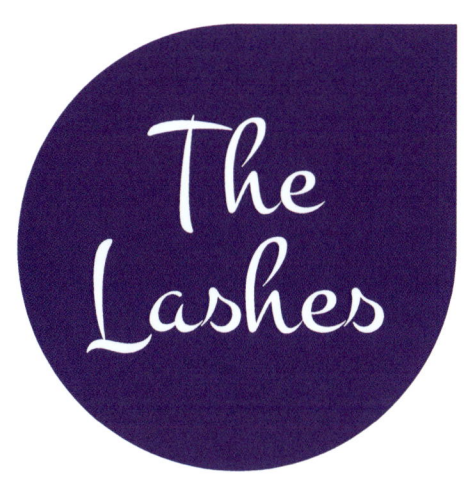
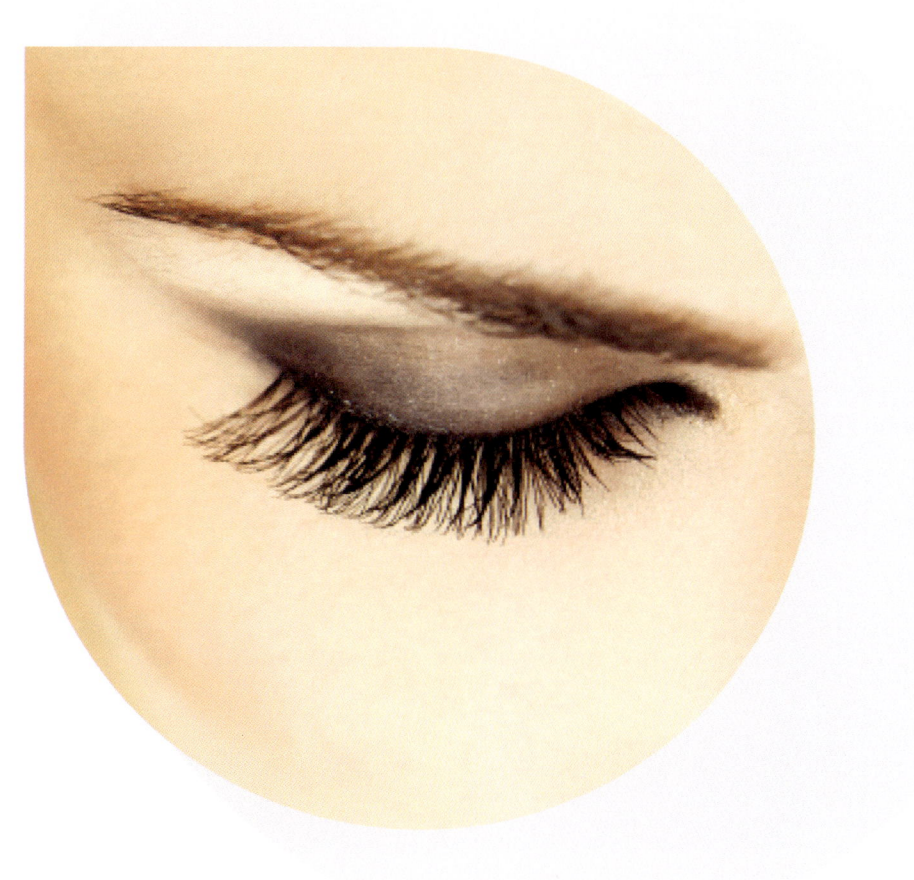

Types

Mink

The thinnest and most lightweight eyelash extensions are real Siberian mink fur that has been gently harvested by combing. Mink is more expensive than the other options and takes more training and practice to apply. They last longer, have less rules and can be used in paramedical eyelash extension application. Our True Sable extensions are gently harvested and cruelty free.

Silk

Premium eyelash extensions are single thread silk fibers that are smooth and glossy to the touch. The silk fibers add the volume and will maintain curl, and are more lightweight and flexible than polyester fiber eyelashes. Many competitors market silk as faux-mink. At Fringe Beneyefits, we want only the best for our clients so we only sell Silk and Mink lashes.

Poly

Heavier, stiffer extensions tend to be made with a single polyester fiber thread. Polyester eyelashes are thick and hold a curl. They are also the cheapest option. They are known for breaking the client's natural eyelashes even when applied correctly because they are not soft and flexible. Not only are they rigid but their weight is an issue as well and can also be a concern for damaging the eyelash hair follicle, sometimes permanently.

Sizes

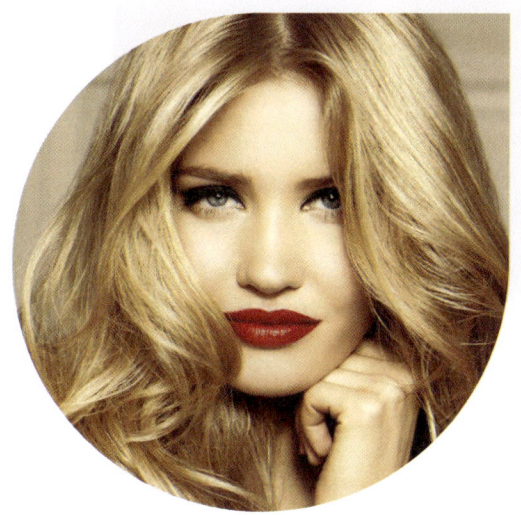

Photo by Betsy Jons

Understanding the different sizes of eyelashes is key to being successful.

All labels come with a formula that looks like this:_____ x _____ mm

The first number you see is the thickness of the eyelash extension and second number is the length of the eyelash extension in millimeters.

Thickness in mm— .07 .10 .12 .15 and .20

.25 and .30 are also available, but not recommended. They are so large they might break your client's natural lashes.

Length in mm— 6 to 17

Again longer lashes are available, but not recommended. I tried 20 mm lashes and they broke my normal strong natural eyelashes.

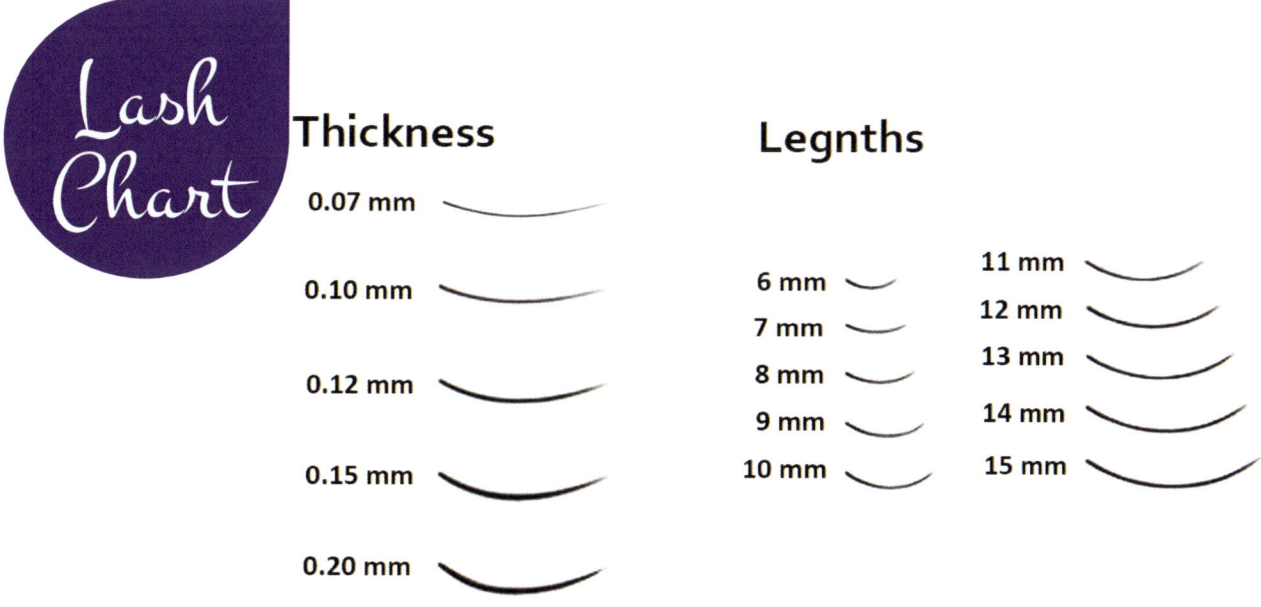

Rules of Sizing Lashes

#1
You can double the natural eyelash length when using a similar thickness to the client's natural eyelash thickness. If you want longer extensions, you can get away with 2 mm longer than double if you go thinner in thickness.

#2
If you want thicker eyelash extensions you will need to use shorter in length extensions.

Usually 6mm is the smallest length you will need to use. I have cut the extension from the base to make it even smaller. If you cut extensions, always trim before application from the thicker base as they are tapered at the end to look like natural lashes. The longest we carry at Fringe Beneyefits is 17mm. I tried 20mm and it broke my thick, strong natural lashes. As the industry grows there are more and more options. I am a huge fan of experimentation. But I suggest always try anything new on yourself or a loved one that will understand you are experimenting and love you unconditionally.

Remember, the first number is thickness and the second number is length in millimeters.

For a natural look go 1-4 mm longer than what they have naturally. Start with smaller eyelashes in the inner corners, then longer throughout. For more dramatic looks, you can use longer extensions. Always consider where her eyebrow is in relation to her lid because you don't want the extension to go up into or above her eyebrows.

**Remember: Extensions are sterile in the jars.
Proper handling of jars with sterile tweezers will eliminate any cross-contamination.**

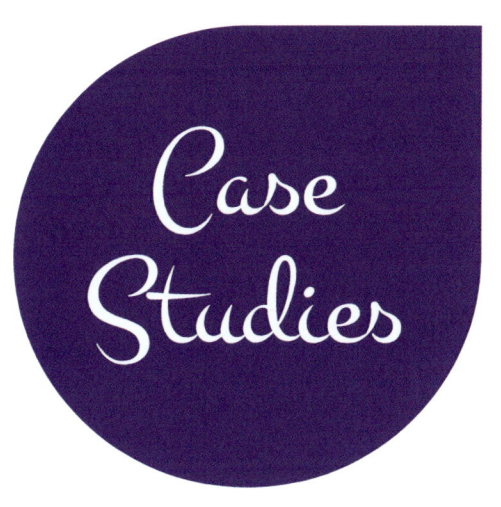

Case Studies

#1 Longer Lashes

Lindsey has healthy eyelashes that are 6mm long. You can use (.15mm x 12mm) eyelash extensions as the longest, doubling her natural length. She requests even longer.

You can use .10 x 14mm extensions because you went with a smaller thickness (.15mm to .10mm) while going longer in length (12mm to 14mm).

#2 Thicker Lashes

Tori has healthy eyelashes that are 7mm long and desires a look that mimics mascara. She says she's not concerned with length as much as fullness.

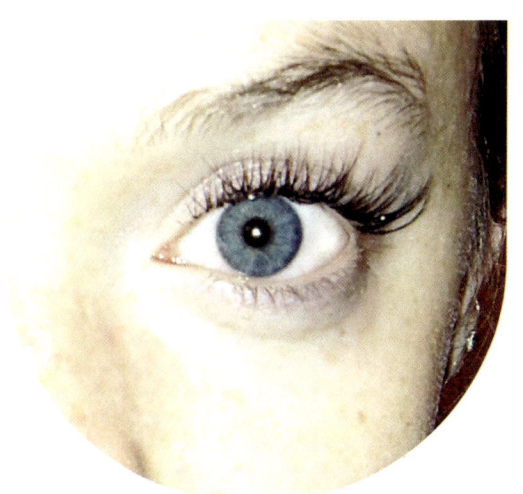

She has healthy lashes that can support the length up to 14mm with the normal .15 thickness. But when using a thicker eyelash, it is going to weigh more and you won't be able to go as long. With Tori you would want to max out at .20 x 13mm. A good mascara look will be 2-3 mm longer than natural so with Tori, use .20 x 9 and .20 x 10.

You will know you have gone too heavy (which can be attributed to thickness or length) if you notice the extensions hanging below her natural eyelash line. Look to the left at the middle of the model's eye. It looks like they almost dip a little blocking the top of her eyeball. This is a very little dip, but it's noticeable to experts like us. Try a shorter or thinner eyelash extension.

Note: If she is coming in for a fill and there has been grow out that causing the extension to hang down lower like the model above, ask the client how long it's been like this. If it's only been a day or two or she hasn't noticed it, I wouldn't worry about it. With extensions there are lots of judgment calls, go with your gut.

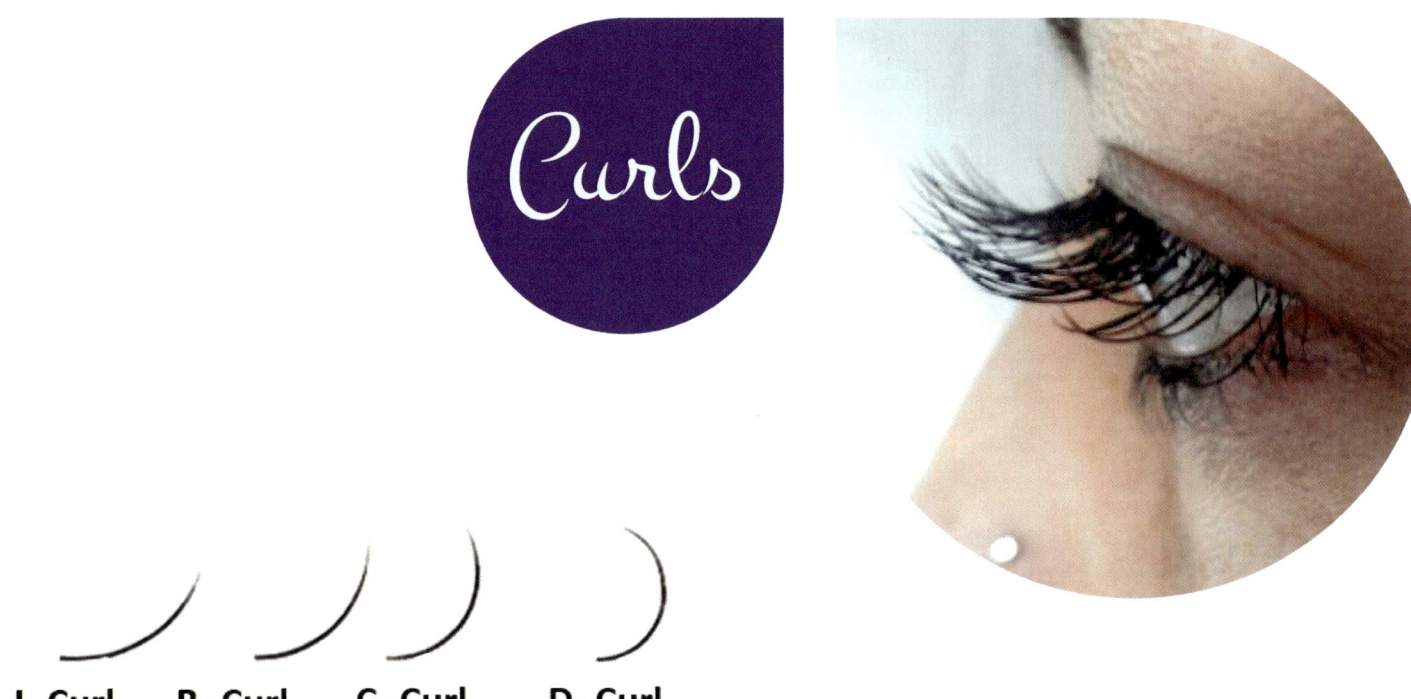

Curls

J- Curl   B- Curl   C- Curl   D- Curl

J- Curl

Most common and most naturl looking curl. For a long time, it was the only option on the market. J-curl is best for most clients.

C- Curl

With an added dramatic curl that stays put, this is a great choice for clients who say they want their eyes to appear more open. It's great for hooded and drooping eyelids as well when you choose a length that goes up over the fold of the lid. When clients want drama or glamor, choose this curl.

Other Curls

For this training we will focus on using the J and C curls. There are a wide variety of curls and once you get going you may want to experiment.

Keeping Lashes Curled

Never under any circumstances use normal eyelash curlers on eyelash extensions. It will break the glue bonds and possibly break the natural eyelashes. Heated eyelash curlers can be used. They are wands that heat up and pop the root of the natural lash up and curl it slightly. Using a blow dryer on the lowest setting can have the same effect. Hold the blow dryer at your waist and point it up towards your face. Gently comb through the eyelashes using a clean mascara wand and POP! Up they go.

Glasses and Glamor

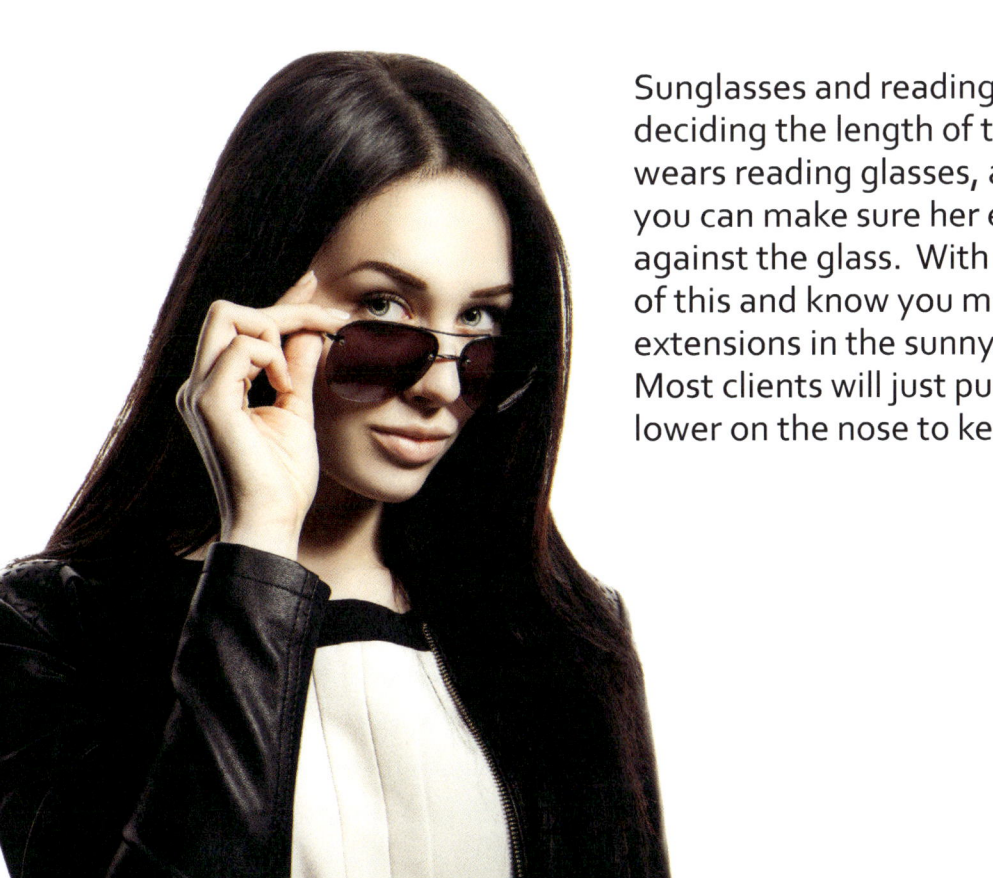

Sunglasses and reading glasses are a concern when deciding the length of the eyelashes. If your client wears reading glasses, ask her to bring them so you can make sure her extensions do not press up against the glass. With sunglasses, just be aware of this and know you may need to shorten her extensions in the sunny months if it bothers her. Most clients will just pull the sunglasses a little lower on the nose to keep their length.

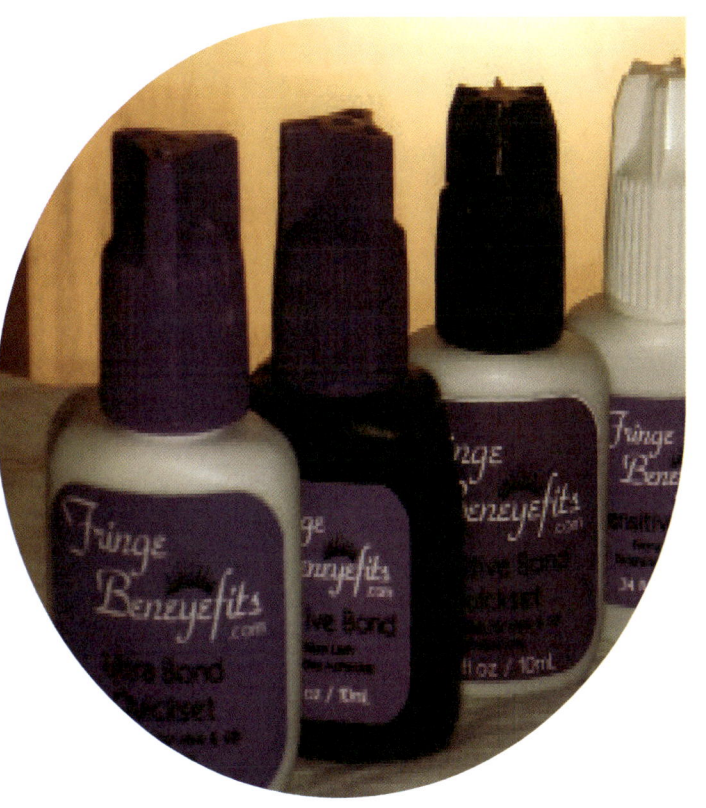

Glues
(Adhesives)

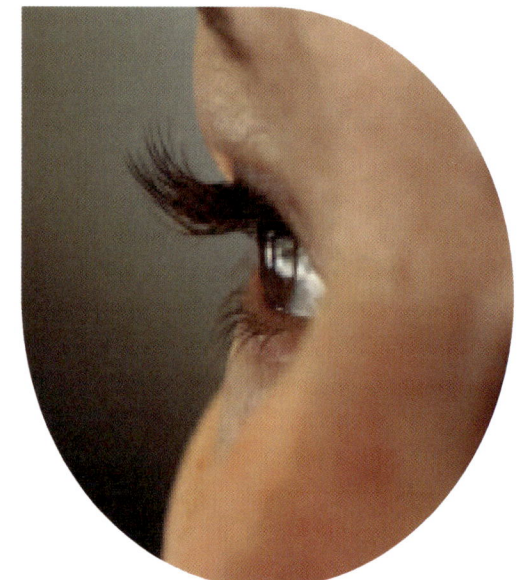

Our glues are designed to be strong, pretty and flexible. We comply with all FDA regulations. Cyanoacrylates have a mild acrid odor while setting. The fume can irritate some people so proper ventilation is needed. This type of adhesive is an irritant if it contacts the skin, eyes or mucus membrane. For this reason, the base of the eyelash extension should always be kept approximately 1mm (the width of a dime) away from the actual eyelid.

Properties of Cyanocrylate

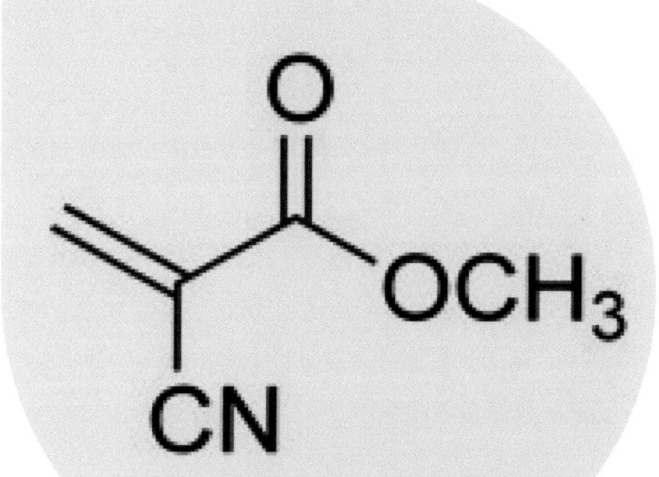

Cyanoacrylate is the generic name for a family of fast-acting adhesives with industrial, household, cosmetic, and medical uses. They include methyl 2-cyanoacrylate, ethyl-2-cyanoacrylate (commonly sold under trade names like "Super Glue" and is also what is used now instead of stitches to glue skin together in emergency rooms.)

Cosmetic grade chemical makeup: n-butyl cyanoacrylate and 2-octyl cyanoacrylate (also used in medical, veterinary and first aid applications).

Octyl cyanoacrylate was developed to address toxicity concerns and to reduce skin irritation and allergic response.

Glue Basics

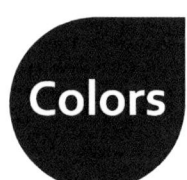

Colors

Quality eyelash extension adhesives are flexible, lightweight, and have a mild acrid odor. They come in two colors, black and clear. Black is best for black and very dark colored extensions. Black is recommended for most applications. Clear is used for lighter colored extensions only.

Careful application is important because adhesives can irritate skin, eyes, and other mucus membranes. Stay away from harsh adhesives.

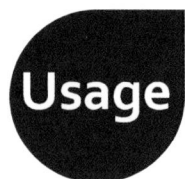

Usage

Adhesives are good for about 6-9 months before opening. After opening they are good for up to 3 months. Store the glue in a cool dark place and mark the date opened for best results. Do not store in the refrigerator. Keep the top clean so the pressure cap doesn't glue to the bottle. Adhesives are 'water adverse'. Over time water will break down glue bonds. Sealants are suggested to enhance the longevity of the bond.

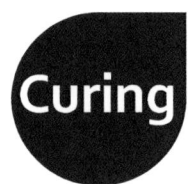

Curing

Eyelash extension adhesive cures in 24 hours by absorbing moisture from the air. Too much water such as a full face of water in the shower, being submerged in a swimming pool or spending an excessive amount of time in a steam room or sauna would be bad for the glue. Avoiding these activities for 24 hours is recommended.

The adhesive can also react with the water vapors in the air and cause blooming. If you see little white crystals on the cap of your glue bottle do not be alarmed, just wipe them off. Likewise if your client has spent too much time in the shower or has had a good cry, you may notice a white film on some extensions. Blooming is not at all harmful, but for aesthetic purposes, I'd reccomend removing the extensions affected by blooming and putting fresh ones on.

Making Your Glue Stick

Setting Speed
The Ultra Bond and the Sensitive Glue are thicker and take a longer time to set up.
They are best for learning with because you have more time to separate out lashes.
Some technicians also prefer more time to set up even after they are seasoned.

The Ultra Bond Quickset and the Sensitive Quickset are just that, quick set glues. Usually as soon as you apply the eyelash extension, it immediately adheres to the natural eyelash. You can work much quicker with this glue and there is less chance of neighboring eyelashes sticking to them. Their viscosities are thinner.

Sticking Power
Bonding Strength-when the glue cures the extension should be attached until the natural eyelash falls out. With Ultra Bond glues the bonding strength is 6-8 weeks. In this time, the client will lose all of her natural eyelashes and grow new ones. So the extensions aren't falling off, your client is just naturally shedding her own lashes. Clients usually get 2-3 week fills with Ultra Bond glues. The Sensitive Glue does not have as much sticking power. Clients with sensitive eyes may see more shedding along with natural shedding. Their own eyelashes will not be damaged if the glue has lost its strength. 10-day fills are recommended for Sensitive glues.

Nano Misters
Nano misters are new on the market and cure the adhesive in 30 seconds. By delivering moisture in mist form the tiny water molecules harden the glue immediately. This reduces the fumes and reactions are practically eliminated. Most reactions are to the glue fumes. It is also easier for your client because now she doesn't have her 24 hour wait list for activities such as showering, swimming pools and saunas. The client can blink while using a nano mister to re-hydrate the eyeballs as well.

GLUE TYPE	LASTS
Sensitive	2-3 Weeks
Sensitive Quickset	3-4 Weeks
Clear	4-5 Weeks
Ultra Bond	5-7 Weeks
Ultra Bond Quickset	6-8 Weeks

Removing and Coating Extensions

Primer
Primer is used to clean off the natural eyelashes. It can pick up makeup residue, natural oils, dust and other pollution. Use microbrushes to apply and make sure to use it sparingly. Do not have enough product on the microbrush to drip into the client's eye as it will create an uncomfortable sensation. Use mulitple times if necessary, until microbrush remains clean and white while brushing the eyelashes.

Lash Ready Extension Bond Enhancer
This magic liquid is FOR EXTENIONS ONLY! NEVER APPLY TO NATURAL EYELASHES! Using a Lash Ready wand, apply to the extensions before application and allow 5-10 second to dry. Extensions need to be used within 24 hours or they will need additional applictions. The Bond Enhancer prolongs the life of the eyelash extensions. The coating allows the extension to adhere to the natural eyelash even better.
NOTE: This product is not reccomended for use with sensitive glues as it may cause irritation in sensitive clients.

De-Fringe Adhesive Remover
We use a gel adhesive remover that comes sealed with similar pressure caps as our glues and should be stored and cared for in the same way: in a cool, dark place. The remover is dimethyl ether and is highly effective. It is a potent irritant to skin, eyes and mucus membranes as well as highly flammable. Never use the De-Fringe Adhesive Remover without eyewash and a towel within an arm's length reach. You will want to rinse her eye out immediately should it get into her eye. The gel remover should be applied with microbrushes. A little bit goes a long way. It sometimes takes 10-20 seconds to work, so be patient and do not use too much at once. If you need to do a full removal, separate each eyelid into 6-10 sections and work in those very small sections one at a time. Never cover more than a quarter of the eyelid at once.
NOTE: ALWAYS have eyewash and a towel at arm's length when using any adhesive remover.

Eyelash Extension Sealant
This is a clear liquid coating made of Teflon and provides an effective extra layer of waterproofing. Use it in every application as the last step of the procedure. The client can also take a bottle home and apply it every 2-3 days. Black sealant is also available. If your client is determined to wear mascara, special eyelash extension mascara should be worn in conjunction with the sealant. The mascaras safer for use with eyelash extensions are water-based.

Client Consultation

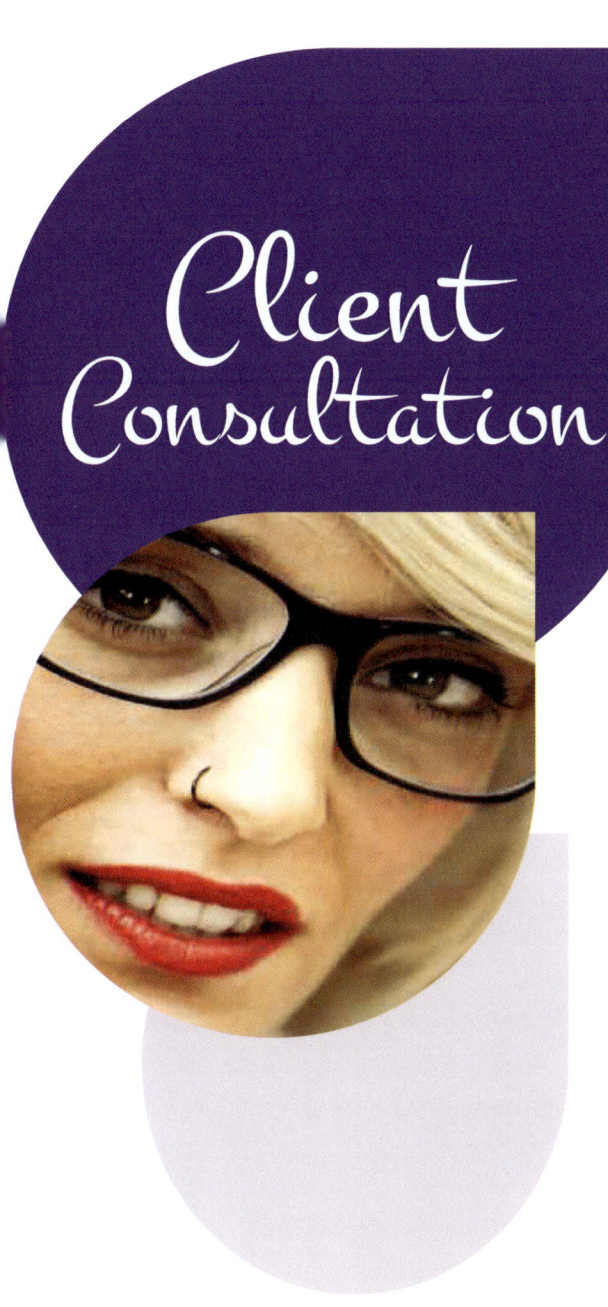

Remember

The consultation is very important. You need to cover every point with every client. Even people you may know well can suprise you with their answers.

Each consultation should include review of the following:

- **Client Care Card**
- **Medical History**
- **Cosmetics and Care**
- **Consent Forms**
- **Understanding Expectations**

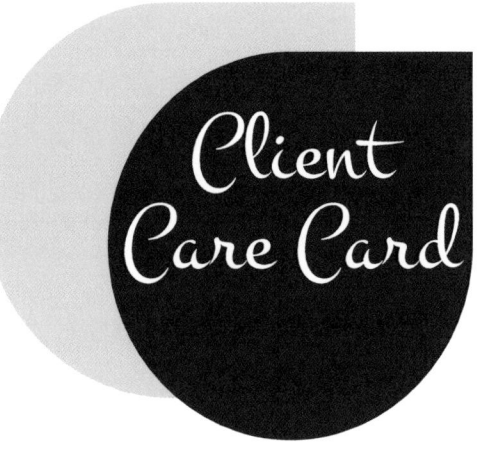

A sample of the client care card is in the back your manual in the appendix. It would be helpful to look at it now as we go over it.

The front of the client care card should be filled out by the client. The back is for you to keep track of services.

Medical History asks if the client is under a doctor's care. This means long term care. If they have a thyroid problem or other hormonal problem that affects hair growth, it can affect the shedding of the eyelashes. Discuss the expectations and let them know they may need fills more often than normal. If they are undergoing chemo therapy, they are not a good candidate for extensions. Since we do not apply extensions to the skin, they lose their extensions if they lose all their natural eyelashes.

The card asks about diabetes and epilepsy as well. You would want to know if your client had the possibility of a low blood sugar coma or seizure since they will be lying down with you for an extended period of time. They are not contraindications.

Accutane and Retin-A are skin thinning medications. Occasionally you may accidently drop an eyelash during application, sometimes on her cheek. If this should happen, the glue and remover has the potential to cause severe damage to the skin. You would want to let them know this is a possibility and even take extra precautions. Drape the face if you decide to take this person as your client.

Smoking and stimulants can make the eyes shaky. You do not want your client to have fluttering lids. Ask her to avoid excessive caffeine before her appointment.

PRO TIP: Each question is important. Gathering the right information will keep you and your client safe and produce the best results.

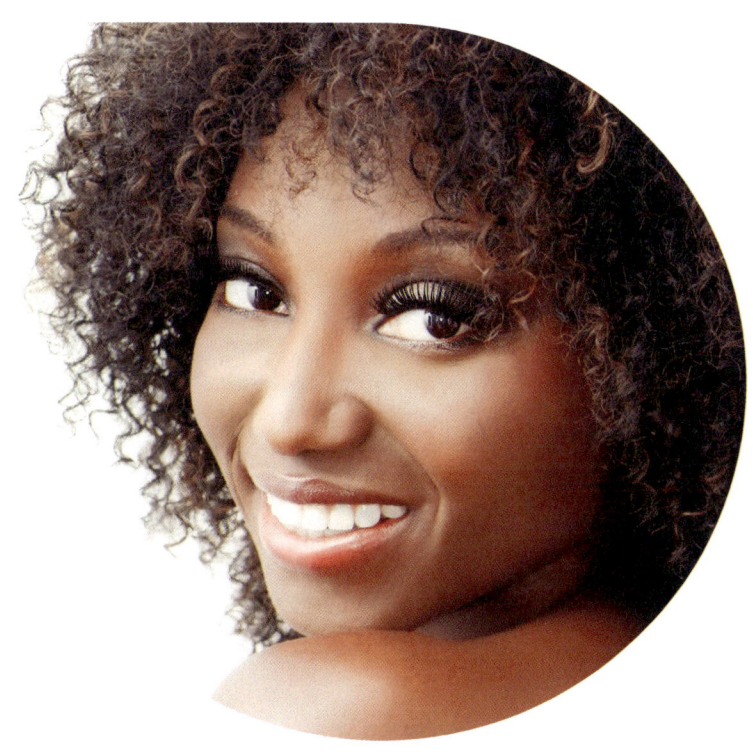

PRO TIP: Gathering all your client's information up front will save you time later on. Not to mention helping you avoid potential serious problems.

Allergies are very important. Usually, food allergies are of no concern. If someone is very sensitive or has multiple allergies, you should do a patch test. I recommend putting about 3 eyelash extensions on the outside corner of her eye. I apply Sensitive glue on one eye and the Ultra Bond on the other. Make her wait 24-48 hours. If she feels puffiness, soreness and/or sees a rash, then obviously extensions are not for her.

Medications that increase light sensitivity and/or affect hair growth. If she has a sensitivity to light you will need to make sure she can lie with her eyes closed without her eyes shaking if you use a spot light. The hair growth has already been explained, what affects hair growth affects the natural eyelashes shedding.

Previous experiences with eyelash extensions. If she's had bad reactions to glue you will want to do a patch test. Do not be talked into doing a full set because "the client thinks it is okay". You are the expert and you know she needs a patch test. Also, pay special attention to how the client talks about the technician she saw. If she's complaining that the other technician didn't make them full enough, long enough, or thick enough but you can see she has thinning or brittle natural eyelashes, you will need to explain the rules of extensions to her and tell her what she can expect from you.

Brands of skincare can help you find culprits with oil if you notice excessive shedding. There is no way for us to know every single brand but just jotting these down will jog your client's memory as well and you can discuss make up removal. Oily products will weaken the glue bond.

Consent Forms

Photo by Dwayne Bent

Consent forms discuss what eyelash extensions are and how long they last.

The forms explain that eyelash extensions do not damage your own natural eyelashes with proper care.

They also contain before and aftercare instructions.

You will be sending her home with an aftercare card. I recommend verbally going over the aftercare. The more times she sees and hears it, the more she will retain it.

A sample of a consent form is in the back your manual in the appendix.

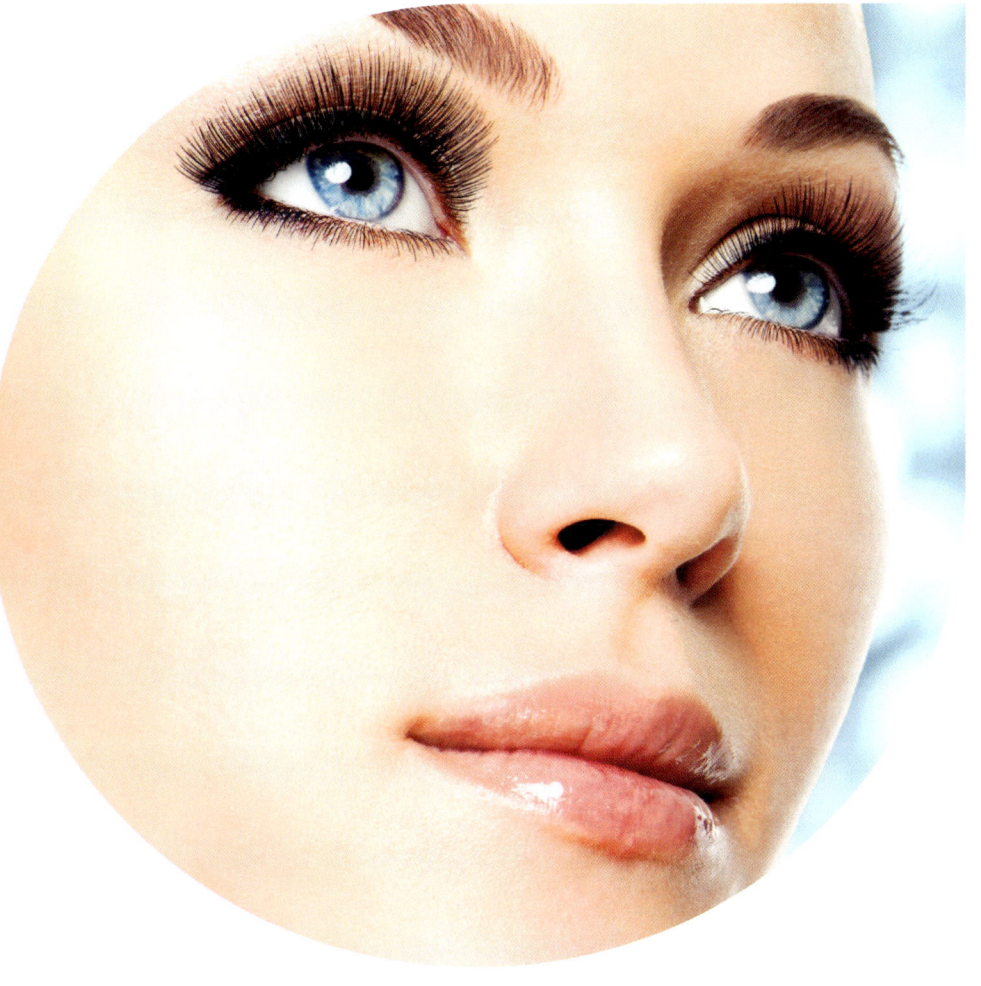

Give Her The Look She Wants

Understanding and setting expectations is critical to client retention and making them happy! Ask her if she wants a natural or glamour look. Does she wear her make-up in a cat-eye? Does she normally wear mascara and how dramatic is it? Ask her why she is getting extensions. These questions will help you determine her look.

Once you have determined she is a good candidate for eyelash extensions, you will want to get started. Some technicians like to take before and after photos. This is a good time to take a photo.

Before and After Photos

Front-eyes open

Front- eyes closed

Profile-Tell them to focus on something straight infront of them so you can see the length of the eyelashes.

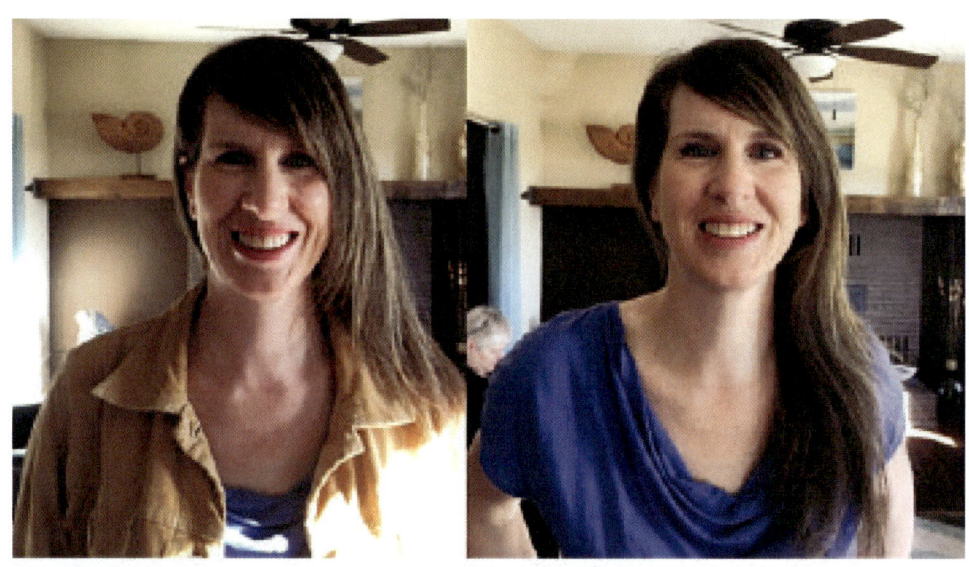

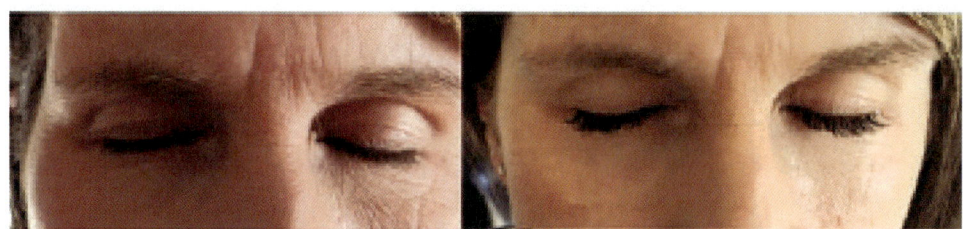

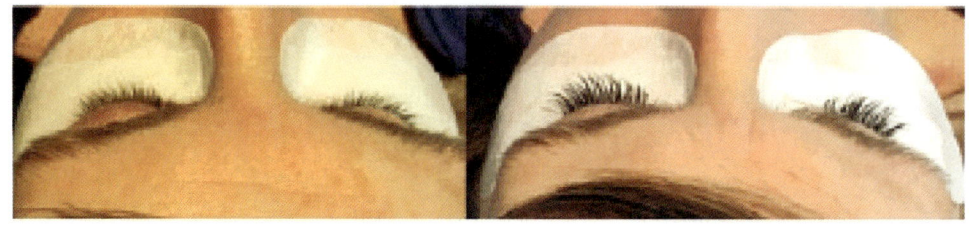

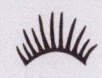

You can never take too many pictures. Your clients will love them and they make great portfolio pieces

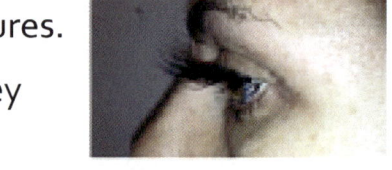

Setting Up the Tray

- 3 Shot Glasses
    - Water
    - Alcohol
    - Acetone - put a cotton ball in this one
- Eyepads
- Paper Tape
    - Pre-cut into four 1.5inch strips
- Plastic Tape
    - Pre-cut into four 1.5inch strips
- 2 Straight Tweezers
- 1 Curved Tweezer
- Sealant
- Fringe Beneyefits Glue
- Lash Ready Bond Enhancer
- De-Fringe Gel Remover
- Primer
- Q-tips
- 2 Microbrushes
- Mascara Wand
- Sealant Brush
- Lash Ready Brush
- Crystal Glue Pallet
- Silicone Eyelash Pad

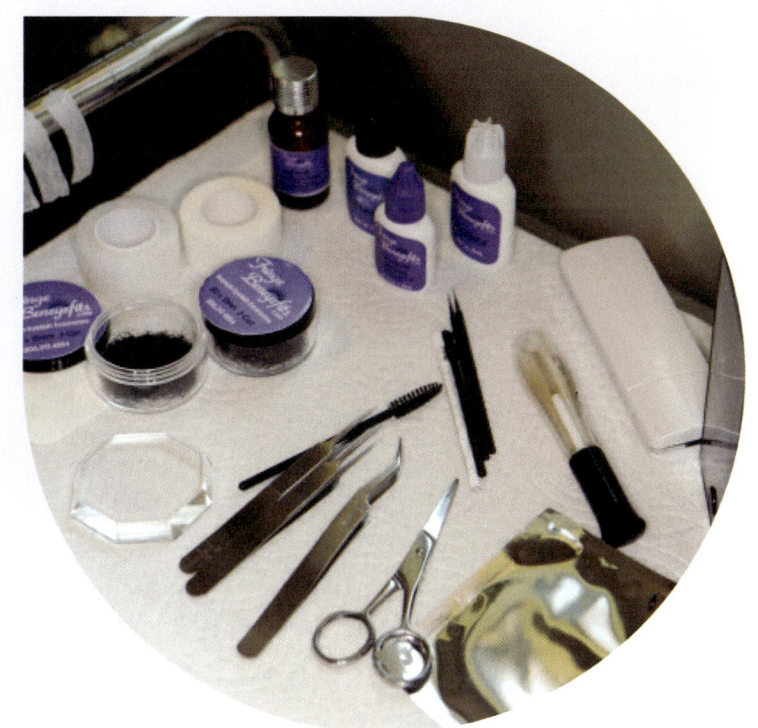

NOTE: We sell mini labels to help you keep track of which clear liquid is which.
NOTE: I put everything on wax paper sheets or paper towels for easy clean-up.

Preparing the Client

Remove Makeup and Contacts
If she wears contacts, ask her to remove them before you get started. You also want to make sure she isn't wearing eye makeup. If she has mascara on you will want her to wash her eyes at a sink. You will want to have washcloths and gentle foaming eyewash remover available.

Taping Lower Lashes
You will want to tape the lower lashes down so there is a barrier between them and the glue on the upper lashes. This prevents you from glueing her eyes shut.

To tape lower eyelashes you will want to put eyepads down first. Eyepads protect the skin from the tape you are about to put on the eyelashes. They should be placed just below the eyelashes or if you have a client with long lower lashes, then on top of them. You do not want the eyepads to touch the waterline.

Next put gentle paper tape down. This tape should go up to the waterline but not cover it. The paper tape is used because it is gentle and will not pull out the natural lashes.

Next use plastic tape. This goes directly on top of the paper tape. Again, make sure you do not cross the water line as you do not want to scratch or otherwise irritate the eyeball.

The plastic tape allows the glue to be easily released if excess touches the tape. Technicians that only use paper will often see little white pieces of paper attached to the underside of the eyelash.

The lower lashes need to be completely covered so if you need to use more plastic tape or start over please do. If your client is having a hard time with this part of the procedure you can have her look up.

NOTE: Some people's faces are shaped in such a way that when they close their eyes the tape and eyepads will push on the upper lashes. Gently move the eyepads lower while her eye is closed. Adjust the eyepads and tape until the plastic tape no longer pushes on the upper lashes. Once this is complete, lift the lid while her eye is closed to make sure there are no lower lashes showing. You may need to re-tape or adjust again.

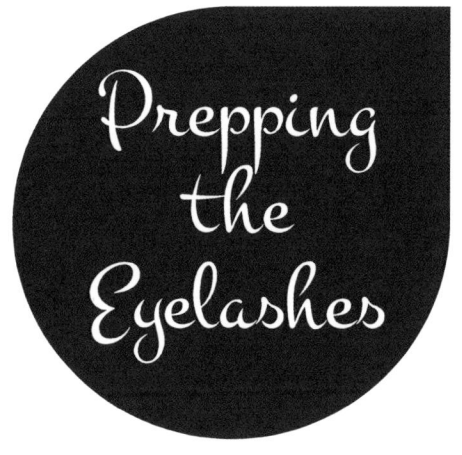

Prepping the Eyelashes

Once she is taped you can have her close her eyes. Let her know that now she needs to keep her eyes shut. The glue fumes will not harm her but if she opens her eyes before you tell her to she will feel a definite burning sensation.

Use primer on the microbrushes to clean each eyelash. Primer is good for removing natural oils and dust from the eyelashes.

If your client has residue mascara, you will want to use q-tips and foaming cleanser to clean off the mascara first. Then use the primer. Likewise if there is glue on the natural eyelashes and no extensions are present, you will want to remove the glue with the remover and then use primer. Keep cleaning until the microbrushes remain white and no longer show any residue.

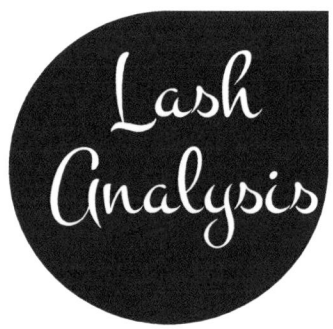

Lash Analysis

You will now look for any signs of disease or irritation in or around the lash line. If she is irritated, do not apply extensions. You will be looking to see if she is a good candidate for eyelash extensions. You will also want to notice:

- **Length and density of the lashes**
- **Shape of lash line-are there any gaps**
- **Does she have multiple rows of eyelashes?**
- **Shape of eyelashes-are they straight, curled, crimped?**
- **How the lash lies- is it naturally crooked or leaning?**
- **What color are her natural lashes?**

These are all great things to note on the front of the client care card. This is a good time to take a before photo at this angle.

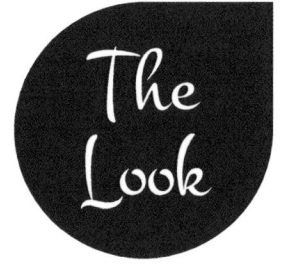

The Look

Now it's time to design the perfect look for your client.

1. Choose the size and curl of the lashes based on the consultation and the look she wants.
2. Pull those jars and take just a few lashes from each jar.
3. Later dip the tweezer in alcohol before reaching in to the jar to prevent cross contamination.

Application

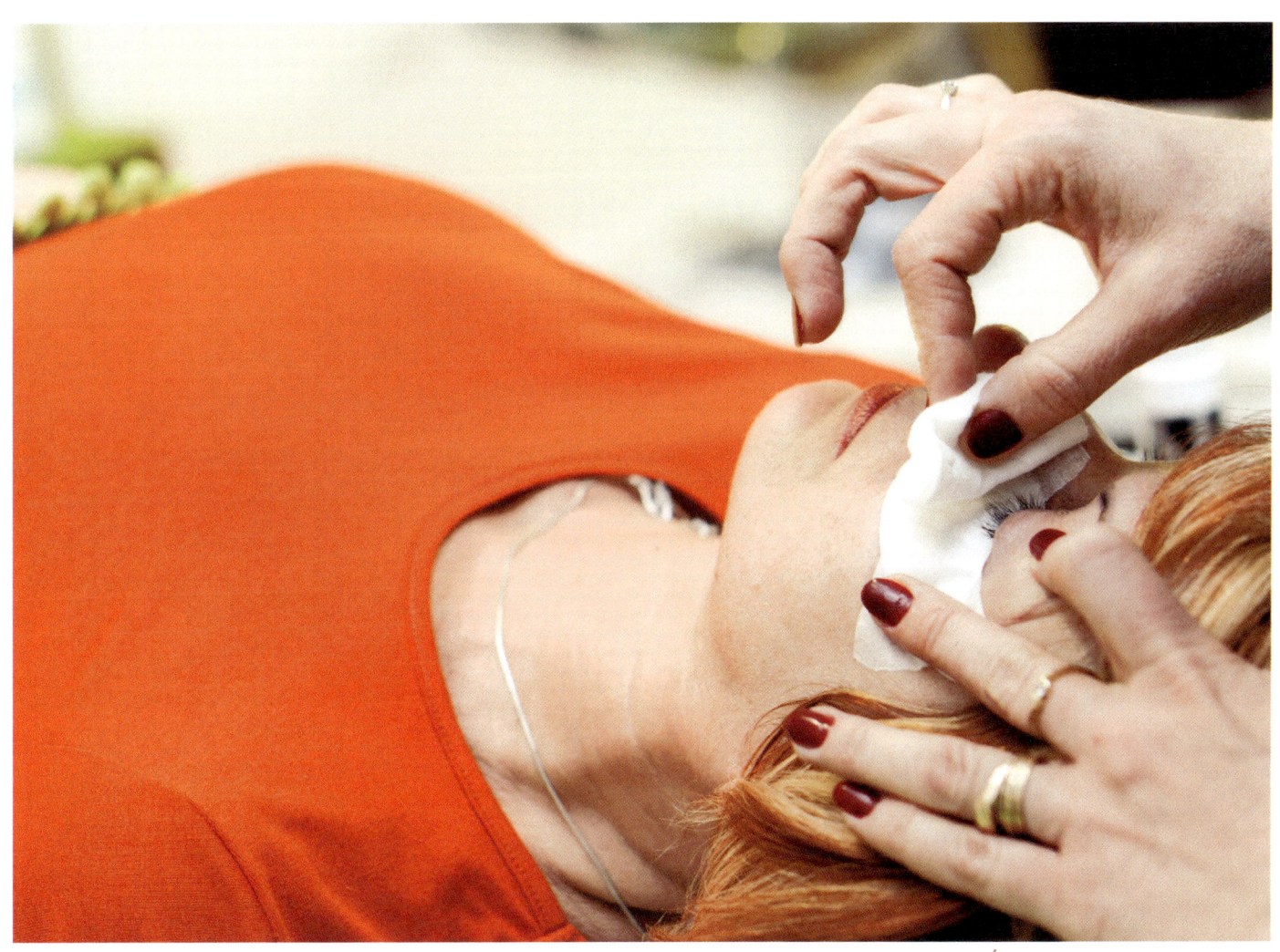

 **Put one pea sized drop of glue on your crystal pallet.** As you work try not to rest your hands or wrists on the clients forehead. She is not your working space or table! Occasionally steadying your hand for balance when needed is acceptable. Many clients complain and will not return if there is too much pressure on her forehead.

 **Dip the extension in glue at the base.** The entire extension does not need to be coated, just the lower half. Estimate the length of her natural eyelash and dip the extension in at that point and slowly draw it through the glue puddle. You should see a tiny ball of glue at the bottom of the extension. That is good. If there is a larger ball or many little balls, touch the extension to the crystal pallet gently to remove excess but be very careful not to remove it all. Over time this will become very easy to do, don't get frustrated.

 **Isolate an eyelash using the curved tweezers.** Separate the lashes until just a single eyelash is isolated. Never put an extension on multiple natural lashes.

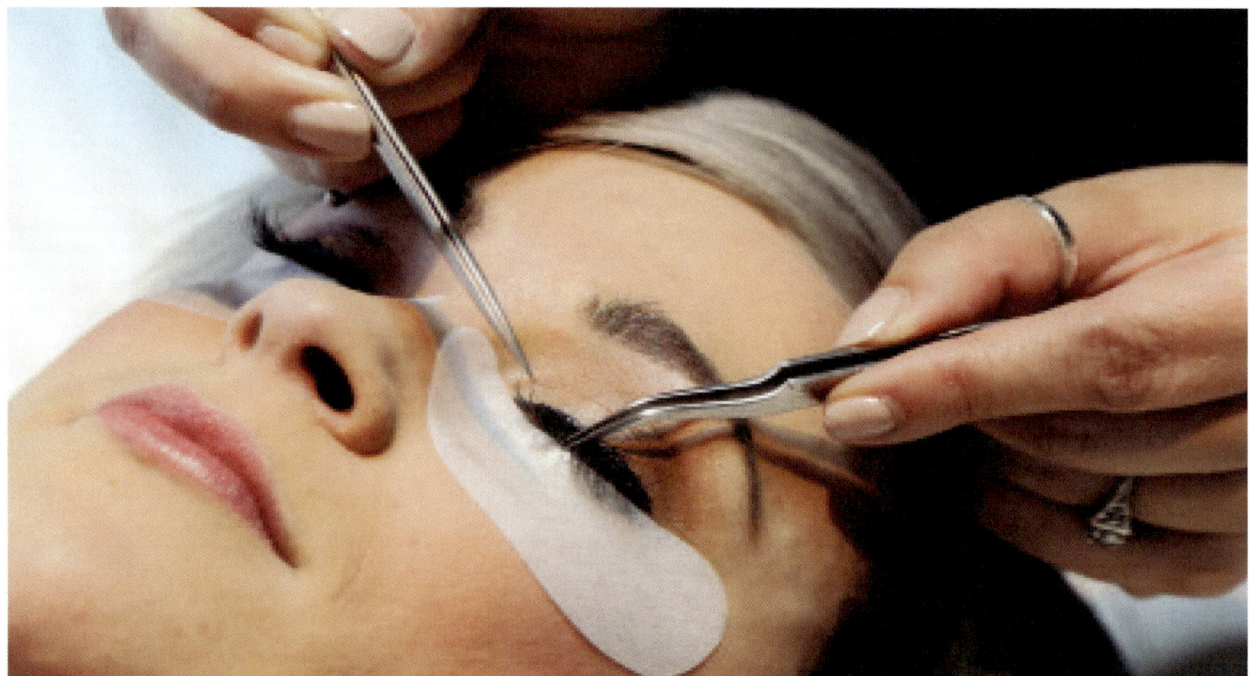

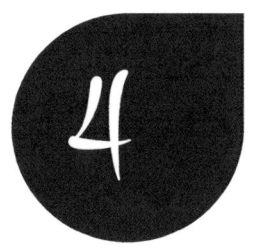

Coat the eyelash with glue and place the extension directly on top of the eyelash 1mm away from the eyelid.
That is about the thickness of a dime. It's as close to the lid as you can get without touching the lid. With the thicker glues, you may need to hold the lash in place for 3-5 seconds before moving on. With the quick set glues, you can place and move immediately. If as you place the lash it leans to one side or the other, use the straight tweezers at the top of the extension to push it back in place. It may not be necessary to pick it up again, just gently push it into place.

If you notice excess glue, gently use the end of a microbrush to absorb the excess. I recommend just barely touching the excess ball. You do not want to brush the entire lash or press very hard because you don't want to take glue away from the extension. You want to prevent clumps and make it look natural. If you are tempted to use your tweezers to remove the excess glue, just be aware you will need to thoroughly clean them before moving on to applying more extensions.

Start at the corner of one eye and do about 4 extensions spaced out, then move to the next eye.
If you work back and fourth this way, you will not see the neighboring eyelashes sticking together. You will also want to periodically comb through the extensions making sure the neighboring natural lashes have not stuck to the glue.

If you do have some "stickies" as I like to call them, use both pairs of straight tweezers. Hold the extension with one set as you pull the natural lash away.

It is is fun and exciting to see the look coming together. If your client has a lot of natural eyelashes you may want to run a fan over her lashes to encourage all the glue to dry and discourage stickies periodically as you go.

Check extensions for full attachment.

If the top is glued but not the bottom, you can hold the natural eyelash with one set of tweezers and then hold the extension at the bottom and gently pull the extension off the natural eyelash, making sure not to pull too hard. Sometimes you can pull from the top but be careful not to pull so hard you crimp the lash or tug on it too hard once it is released. If there is a huge clump, you may want to use the adhesive remover. The extension will come off and you will need to reapply it. Always have eyewash and a hand towel present when using the adhesive remover.

When you think you have all the eyelash extensions placed, you should count how many are on each eyelid.

This will help you see where there are strays and room for more. It will also help you determine if both eyes are even. Make sure you have extensions on the inner and outer corners. Sometimes outer corners will need to be re-taped if the tape has moved during conversation. Make sure to note the number of eyelash extensions on your client care card once you are finished.

A fun tip is to pull the eyelashes back, almost like you are lifting the lid, to find any lashes without extensions that are buried underneath. If they are an acceptable length and not new growth lashes, you can apply an extension. Dental mirrors can also help see the underside of the lash line as well.

The last step of application is to use a sealant brush to apply sealant to each eye's extensions.

Dip the disposable wand into the sealant tube. This will be enough product for both eyes. Do not double dip to avoid cross contamination. Coat each eye at the base of the eyelashes. This is an extra layer of protection. It is Teflon, so it repels water, dust, makeup and whatever else tries to get on the extensions. This is also a great retail take home product for your client.

Taking Off the Tape

Before you take the tape off. Lift each lid slightly to make sure none of the lower lashes has gotten loose and is stuck to an upper lash. Occasionally this will occur. The lash is almost always just barely attached and running the straight tweezers between the lower lash and extension will release it.

If you are stuck. If tweezers aren't working, you may use adhesive remover or small eyebrow scissors. Take note not to use the tweezers or scissors too close to the lids or eyeball itself. Also note that if you use scissors and cut the lower lashes, it may be very noticeable for clients with long lower lashes. If it is going to cause more than one eyelash to be cut, I'd recommend the De-Fringe Adhesive Gel Remover.

Now its time to take the tape off. Remove the plastic tape first and then the paper tape. The client can keep her eyes closed at this time, but there is no harm in opening. Do not take off both sets of tape at once as it is common for the natural lower lashes to get caught in between the two sets of tape. You do not want to pull them out.

Finishing Up

Take before and after pictures. Usually this is best to do both before and after she sits up.

Have the client sit up and open her eyes. I highly recommend sitting up first as the lights will be very bright after so long on the table with eyes closed.

Give her a mirror and watch her smile. You also need to look at her face on to make sure there is no drooping, crazy sideways lashes or any other problems.

Don't be afraid to correct an error if you see it. Your client would rather be taped up again and look perfect. She will appreciate the extra time and effort. Never be in a hurry or rush a procedure. This attention to detail will set you above the competition.

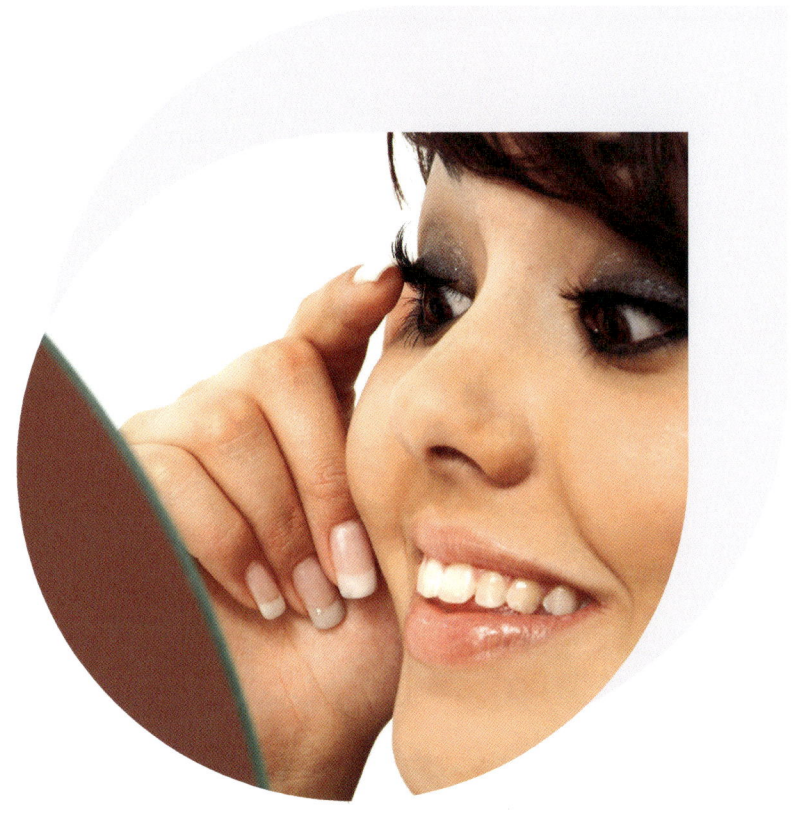

Fill Out the Client Care Card

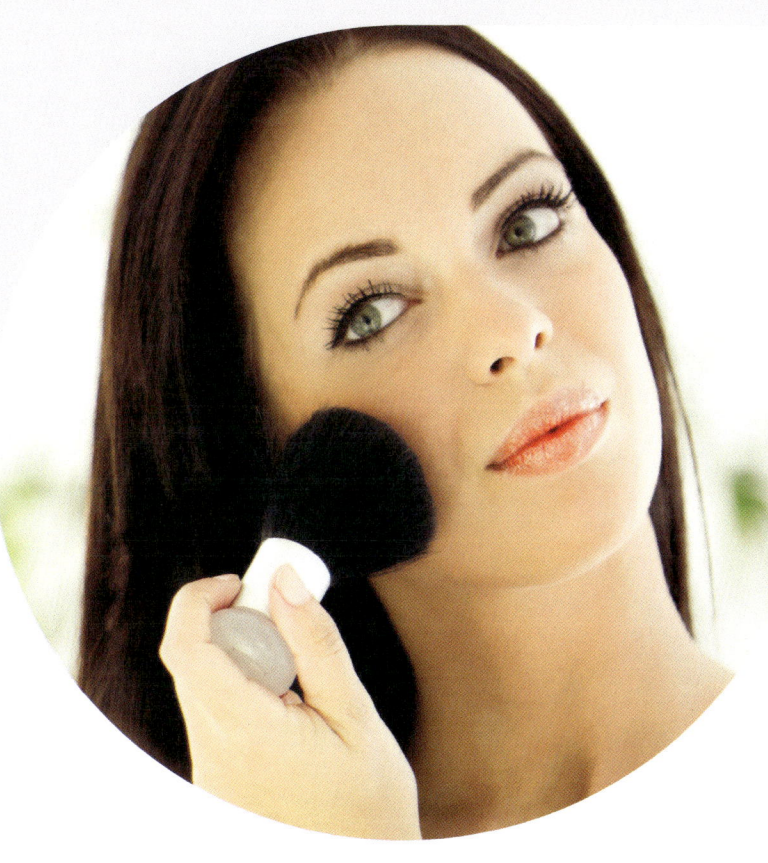

First note the sizes and curl used. In the lid section indicate what sizes were used in each area of the eye.

Next note the number of eyelash extensions you used on each eyelid. On the back of your client care card is a place to write the number down for each eye. This will help you when she comes in next time for a fill.

J-Curl .15 x 9, 10, 11mm   75, 75

This is also a great place to make notes about upcoming events, children's names, etc. This will help jog your memory for conversation that builds rapport.

Read over the instructions for care one last time. It may feel like overkill, but I can't tell you how many clients come back completely bald because they forgot and put an oily product too close to their lashes.

Removing Lashes

Banana Peel Method
Using two straight tweezers, hold the base of the eyelash with one set and the base of the extension with the other. Gently peel off the extension. Holding the natural lash at the base will prevent you from hurting the client by pulling too hard.

If a lash is not grown out or if the extension is not free at the base, you can hold the natural lash at the base with one set of tweezers. Then hold the extension with the other hand and gently press down towards the lid. The extension will release at the base and you will be able to banana peel it off.

Adhesive Remover
If the banana peel method does not work, you will have to use adhesive remover. Have eyewash and a hand towel available. **NEVER, EVER, USE THE REMOVER WITHOUT EYEWASH NEARBY.** Nearby as in an arm's length away. Using two microbrushes, get a very small amount of product and rub the eyelash extension (or glue residue)

It will take 10-20 second for the remover to work. Keep gently working the eyelash, rubbing lightly. Pay special attention not to pull the lid up as you do not want product or fume to get into the eye. Once you are done, use q-tips dipped in water to remove any residue the adhesive remover left.

If you are taking off a whole set or many lashes work in small areas. I would not put remover in multiple locations at once. Divide each eye into 6-10 sections and do them one section at a time.

Always sanitize the tray or surface you are placing the set-up on. If you choose to use wax paper like me for easy clean-up, you still need to sanitize the surface the paper is placed on.

The tweezers always need to be sanitized in a barbicide solution or UV sterilizer. Do not use a barbicide container that you place the tweezers in point down as they will get distorted and not work. Trays work best as tweezers can lie flat.

Throw away any extensions you have not used. DO NOT put them back into the jars as this will cause cross contamination. The tips of your tweezers have been near the clients lashes and then near the extensions on the tray that you didn't use.

In order to prevent waste, take small batches of extensions out of the jars. Before you reach in for more, make sure you dip the tweezer in alcohol and dry it.

If there is excess glue on the tweezers, you can dip it in the acetone and gently rub the glue with the cotton ball in the acetone. Small buffing block files work too. Which ever method you prefer, dip the tweezers in alcohol next and then water.

Throw away all disposables. You can sanitize a mascara brush wand 1-3 times before throwing it away but all other microbrushes, sealant brushes, and q-tips need to be thrown away. Do not re-use these items. Ever.

Never reuse an eyepad on a different client.

NOTE: You can give the mascara wands to your clients for home care.

Fills

Fills are exactly the same as a full sets, except fills have the added steps of evaluation and cleanup.

Evaluation

Before you do anything ask her how her extensions are doing. Some clients want to have a thicker look or change the length. If she complains too many fell out, go over the aftercare again and try to troubleshoot what went wrong. At the end of a fill make sure you note if you've made any changes to size, length or curl of the lash.

Clients can get defensive or even blame the technician. It is common to hear, "you didn't put enough glue on this time" or "you did something different". It is best to use words like "let's troubleshoot this together". You can explain how you use the same amount of glue and the same technique every time. It is most likely she used a new product with oil in it if there is more shedding than normal. We will go over more troubleshooting in just a bit.

Cleanup

After you have consulted the client and taped them, part of the prep will be clean up. You will need to observe her lashes and look for extensions that are not completely attached and remove them. You will look for extensions that have grown out. If there is more than 2mm (2 dime thicknesses) between the lid and the base of the extension, it is best to remove it and reapply a new extension at the base. If there is glue residue on the natural eyelash, it will also need to be removed.

When all removal is done, you will need to count how many eyelash extensions are on each eye. Put that number down on her client card. This will provide a running log of how she is doing in her aftercare. I like to note not only how many remain attached but how many I had to remove. I do this by first putting the number reamaining for example, 42. Then using a minus sign I write the number I removed for example, -4.

My client card will look like this:

42 -4, 45 -4
(Left eye, right eye)

Now its time to use the primer and start the original prep.
If she has less than 10 extensions on either eye, you are basically doing another full set. You can decide how much you will charge for the additional time and product. I would let her know before you start the fill that there will be an additional charge. Some technicians choose to do that fill at the normal rate but let the client know that if it happens again, an additional charge will apply. Your time is valuable, you need to train the clients on how to care for the lashes. You do not want a client that waits until the extensions all fall off 6-8 weeks later to schedule a fill and expect a normal fill price.

Melted Tips
Whether it is opening an oven or getting too close to the BBQ, the tips of the extensions can appear completely crimped. All crimped extensions need to be removed and reapplied.

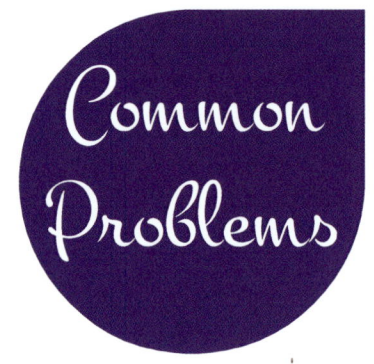

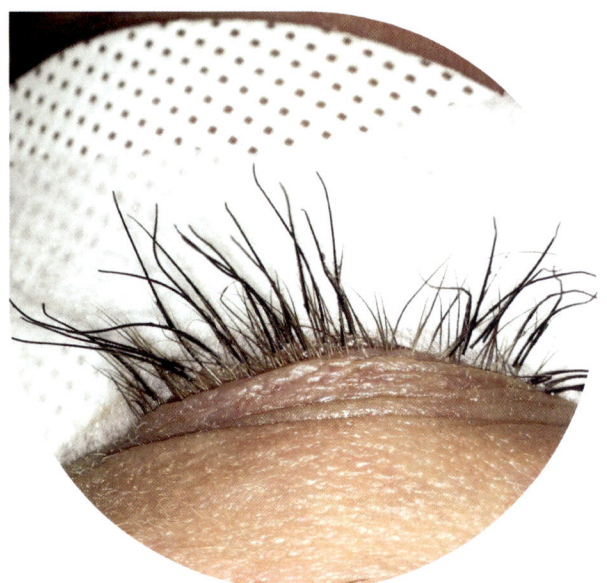

Clumps
Even with our best efforts, occassionaly two neighboring eyelash extensions will stick together. You can separate them using two sets of straight tweezers. If you are cleaning up someone else's mess and you have multiple natural lashes or extensions stuck together, sometimes it is just easier to use the adhesive remover.

Allergic Reaction to the Adhesive
Small red dots (rash) or puffy pink swollen skin at the lids is the most common indication of a reaction to the glue. If there is minor pinkness or she is complaining of being sore, you can remove and reapply extensions using the sensitive glue. If there is major pink skin, broken skin or a rash of any kind, I recommend complete removal and healing of the skin before any more application. Have the client come back in when she's better and do the patch test with sensitive glue on each side. If you prefer using the Sensitive Quickset but have a very sensitive client, consider the regular Sensitive, but do the patch test with both. The Senstive on one eye and the Sensitive Quickset on the other. The Sensitive is the least reactive glue.

Gaps in the Natural Lash Line
There can be gaps from surgery, injury or just natural growth. You can use the stacking method to cover the gap with mink extensions but I don't recommend it with synthetic. If you are going to try with synthetic please use the .07 extensions. With mink, because they are so lightweight, you can have more than one extension per natural lash, even when they are short. On either side of the gap, you can put an extension on as usual and another slightly crooked to cover the gap. The stacking method is covered in detail in Advanced Techniques training.

If the gaps are new and come up during a fill, you need to problem solve why. If it's allergy season or she has had a good cry, she may have been rubbing them and pulled them out. Some people are pickers. They twist and pull on their eyelashes out of nervousness, like someone biting their fingernails. The worst reason would be if the extensions are too heavy or too long and the natural eyelash has been pulled out. We of course would never have applied extensions improperly, but you need to be aware of this option if someone else's client comes to you for help.

Seasonal Allergies
If it is allergy season I recommend a consult on trying not to rub her eyes as much.

Rubbing
If it was a good cry, she really scrubbed/rubbed her face, or any other reason, let her know there is a gap, but not to be alarmed. The natural lashes will grow back. I had a nurse who had an incident where she really needed to scrub her face at work and she came back to me three days later with no extenions attached.

If she is rubbing out of nervousness, consult with her about this. Explain that if she continues to pick, she will not be a good candidate for extensions. The last thing you need is someone blaming you, the technician, because they do not follow instructions.

Too Long or Heavy
If there is no other reason, you may have pushed the limits of length or thickness. Try a smaller extenion. Her eyelashes are not holding the weight of the current extensions. If you think the lashes are too thick or too long, tell the client why you will be using thinner or shorter extenions in her fill.

Good Glue Goes Bad
Keeping track on the client care cards is very important, because if you notice a trend of every single client is coming in with far less extnsions than they normally do, your glue has probably expired. Remember to keep track of it somehow and toss it after 3 months and order a new bottle.

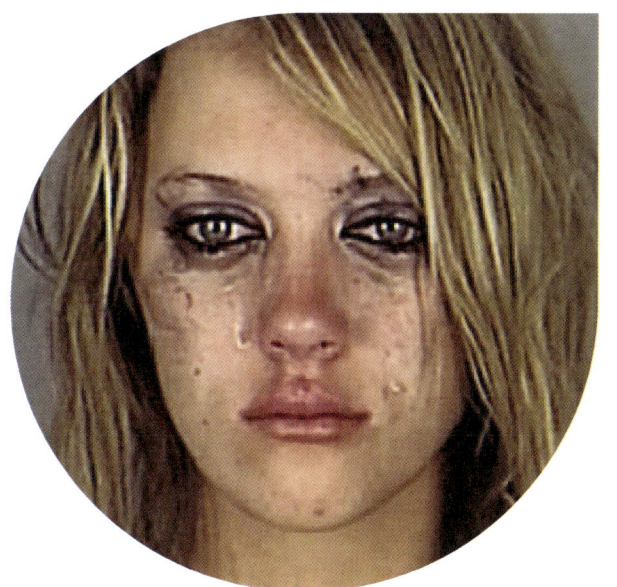

Shedding cycles
I had a client come in once every 2 months with significantly more shedding than usual with no explanation. It was about every 8 weeks. I think her body was just going through a shedding cycle.

Every Other
If you do fills every two weeks and notice a pattern. One week it takes 40 minutes because she only shed 1/4 of her eyelashes. The next visit takes 75 minutes because 3/4 of her eyelashes have shed. This client might say, "it was really good the last time, but this time you must not have put enough glue on". That is not the case. This happens because the majority of the first fill's eyelashes are shedding around the third week. Try extending the fill to 3 weeks to synchronize the fills with her natural shedding cycle. Explain to your client why you think 3 week fills will be better.

How much should I charge?

Setting your price is always tricky at the beginning. If you set it too high, you will not attract new customers. If you set it too low, then it will be harder to raise it later on and you might lose customers. I have found setting the price as high as you want to charge ($250) and then

Be sure to consider the following:

Location and Time Value
Initial Service Costs
Touch up Costs
Test Trial/Consultation Costs
Corrections Costs
Removals Costs

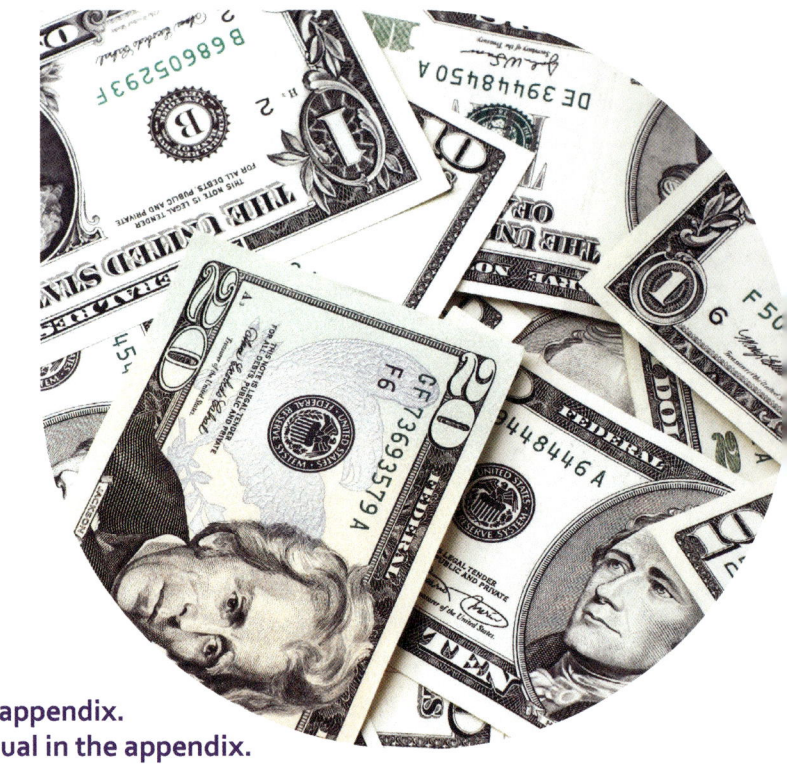

A sample of a menu is in the back your manual in the appendix.
A sample of a industry special is in the back your manual in the appendix.
A sample of an introductory offer is in the back your manual in the appendix.

Do's and Don'ts

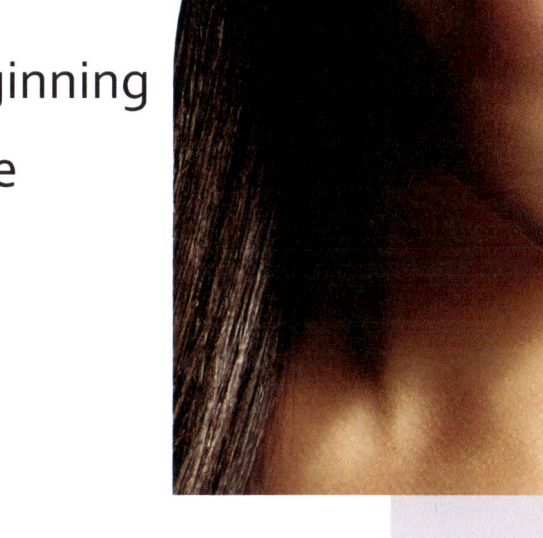

Do Go slow in beginning
Do Take your time

Don't Clump
Don't Put glue on eyelid skin
Don't Use too heavy/long
Don't Stack silk extensions
Don't Forget tape
Don't Cut a bunch of lower natural lashes
Don't Discount your services or time too much

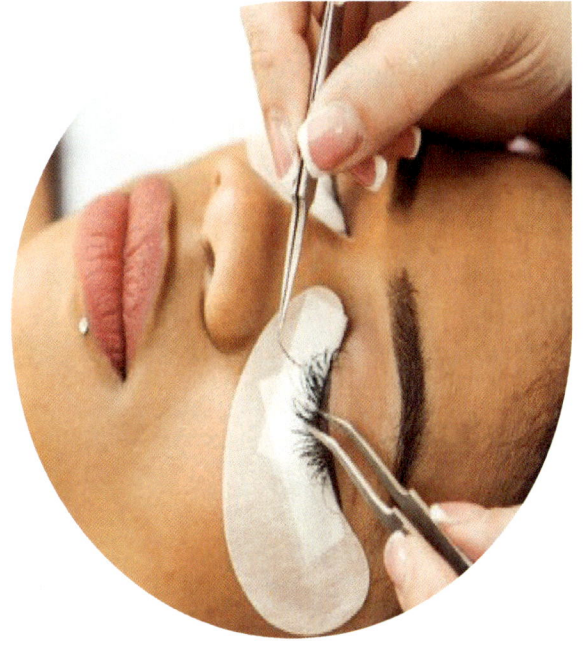

Conclusion

This concludes your Fringe Beneyefits basic training of eyelash extensions. Together we covered how eyelash extensions work and eyelash extension materials and sizing. Next we went over adhesives and specifically our five Glues, Primers, De-Fringe Adhesive Remover and our newest addition Lash Ready Extension Bond Enhancer. Consent forms and proper set-up rounded out the training and got you ready for application. After covering full sets and fills we wrapped up with commonly seen problems and the do's and don'ts of eyelash extensions as well as a discussion of pricing for your clients. I have full confidence that you are now extremely prepared to start your career as an eyelash extension technician. Take it slow and do things correctly and always error on the side of caution.

Once you feel secure in your ability to properly apply extensions I will see you again in the Fringe Beneyefits Advanced Techniques and Advanced Mink classes.

Appendix

Fringe Beneyefits

name:_____ date:_____

phone:(_____)_____ email:_____

address:_____

city:_____ state:_____ zip:_____

How did you hear about us?

Are you currently or within the last year under any doctor's care? If so, please explain.
_____
_____
_____

Have you undergone any recent surgeries? If so, please explain.
_____
_____
_____

Circle all health problems.
Diabetes, Thyroid, Heart, Cancer, Hysterectomy, Hormone Imbalance, Epilepsy, Other:_____

Circle all that apply:
Retin-A   Accutane   Smoking   Stimulants

Do you have allergies or sensitivities to cosmetics, creams, metals, foods, animals, adhesives or other? If so, please explain.
_____
_____
_____

Are you on any medications that increase light sensitivity and/or effect hair growth? Explain.
_____
_____
_____

Have you ever had eyelash extensions before? If so, did you have any reactions?
_____
_____

Please circle your reason for visiting.
Consultation   Full Set   Touch Up   Lash Repair   Lash Removal   Other:_____

Do you wear contact lenses? _____   Are you wearing them today? _____

Have you ever had any surgical or aesthetic procedure(s) around your eyes, such as a facial peel, lash perming or tattoo? If so, please explain.
_____
_____

Please provide brands of personal skin care you are currently using.
Cleanser:_____   Toner:_____   Scrub:_____
Moisturizer:_____   Mask:_____   Eye Makeup:_____
Makeup Remover:_____   Eye Cream:_____   Sunscreen:_____
Treatments:_____   Other(s):_____

Aesthetician's Remarks:_____
_____
_____
_____
_____
_____

All forms are downloadable at www.FringeBeneyefits.com

Fringe Beneyefits

client:_____ phone:_____

date	services	sizes	fee	products	next appt.	aesth. int.

Eyelash Extensions Agreement and Consent Form

Full Name: _____
Telephone: (Cell)_____
Email: _____
Referred by: _____

Initial

_____ I authorize my Fringe Beneyefits trained professional,_____
_____(Professional Name, Business Name) to perform the semi-permanent eyelash extension procedure.

_____ I understand that this procedure requires single synthetic eyelashes to be glued to my own natural eyelashes.

_____ I understand that it is my responsibility to keep my eyes closed and be still during the entire procedure, until my eyelash technician addresses me to open my eyes. This can take from one up to three hours.

_____ I understand that some risks of this procedure may be but not limited to eye redness and irritation. The fumes from the adhesive may cause my eyes to tear up if I open my eyes.

_____ I agree to disclose any allergies that I may have to acrylics, latex, surgical tapes, cyanoacrylate, Vaseline, etc.

_____ I understand that I am required to follow the eyelash extension care sheet (attached)   in order to maintain the life of these extensions.

_____ I agree that by reading and signing this consent form, I release _____
_____(Professional Name, Business Name) from any claims or damages of any nature.

_____ I agree that I read and fully understand this entire consent form and am of sound mind and fully capable of executing this waiver for myself.

_____ I give _____(Professional Name, Business Name) permission to show my before and after photos of eyelashes to other potential clients   Yes _____ or No _____

_____ I have read and completed the Eyelash Extensions Agreement & Consent form in its entirety, and have answered everything to the best of my ability. I have been informed of potentially harmful or negative side effects that may be caused by the application and/or removal of Eyelash Extensions.

I confirm and agree that I wish to engage the services of _____
_____(Professional Name, Business Name)to apply eyelash extensions.

Print Your Name: _____ Signature _____
_____ Date _____

Eyelash Extensions Agreement and Consent Form

What are Eyelash Extensions?
Eyelash Extensions are individual synthetic material. They are attached to your eyelash individually not to the skin. Each synthetic extension is attached to an eyelash. It is a very enhancing beauty service and you DO NOT need to use any mascara while wearing these eyelash extensions. It is a very careful and intense service which requires skill and precision. Once applied these lashes are so natural looking it is difficult to tell even up close that you have extensions on. Size availability ranges from short to long. ___ (initial)

How long do the Eyelashes last?
It is an individual process. We lose at least one eyelash almost everyday. We also grow a new lash to replace the one that fell out. These eyelash extensions can stay on up to 2 full months with proper care and maintenance. However, factors such as eyelash growth, lifestyle and general after care will affect how long the lashes last. Please do not attempt to remove any lashes on your own, seek professional help from your technician. WE WILL NOT BE HELD LIABLE FOR ANY DAMAGE THAT YOU MAY CAUSE BY TRYING TO REMOVE THE EYELASH EXTENSIONS ON YOUR OWN. ___ (initial)

What happens if a lash should loosen or become dislodged?
Do not pull on the lash. Please contact your technician to make an appointment to have them removed or replaced, to avoid damage to your natural lash. As your natural lashes fall out due to the growth cycle, you will need refills when new lashes grow. Most people find fills every 2 weeks to be ideal. _____ (initial)

Do the False Eyelashes damage my natural Eyelashes?
No, not at all! The professional adhesive is formulated to create a solid bond, specifically for human eyelashes. The adhesive dries very soft on the lashes, allowing the lashes to stay flexible and bouncy just like your own natural eyelashes. _____ (initial)

Eyelash extensions are not for everyone. This is a very high maintenance beauty treatment. It requires very gentle care in order for the lashes to last long and stay in good condition. Once the extensions are attached you must not rub or pull on them. It is advised you not wear any mascara. If you must, use water-based mascara. There is mascara especially formulated for eyelash extensions. Never use regular eyelash curlers, as it will break your natural lash and the glue bond. Talk to your eyelash extension technician about more curl or use a heated eyelash curler that is in the shape of a wand. You should read and understand all the information listed below, and sign the form before you get this service done. ___ (initial)

Before Your Appointment
What you should do before your Eyelash Extension appointment. Remove all eye makeup and clean your lashes with mild, oil free cleanser. Do not use oil based makeup removers to clean your lashes prior to the application. Do not put on any mascara. We don't want to spend time cleaning your lashes. We'd rather spend time working on perfecting your lashes. If you are a contact lens wearer, please remove contact lenses and wear glasses to your appointment, or bring a lens case and remove them when you arrive at your appointment. Plan to set aside 1 to 3 hours for your appointment. Some of our clients fall asleep during the procedure. ____ (initial)

Eyelash Extension Information

Your lash extensions are attached to your own individual eyelashes, and will shed as your natural lashesshed. Maintaining your lash extensions will require regular visits to attach new extensions (fills) toyour own eyelashes as your eyelash growth cycle regenerates new lashes.

With a few easy aftercare instructions you will be on your way to enjoying your beautiful lashes. Toincrease the longevity of your extensions, it is advised to avoid moisture and touching as much as possible.

Before your appointment
- If you use waterproof mascara, avoid using it 2-3 days before your first appointment. The film it
leaves on your lashes may prevent the extensions from adhering correctly.
- Arrive to your appointment with dry, clean lashes and makeup-free eyes.
- Remove contact lenses before your appointment.

During the initial 24-48 hours after your appointment
- Do not get your lashes wet for 24 hours after the lash extensions are applied. It will affect the efficacyof the glue.
- Avoid steam from showers, facials, saunas and swimming pools.
- Avoid getting moisture around the eye area when washing face, showering etc.
- Avoid tanning beds for 48 hours after application.
- Avoid chemical peels or laser treatments around the eyes.

General guidelines to extend the life of your extensions
- Avoid using oil-based skincare and makeup products around the eye, including mascara and makeup remover.
- Avoid waterproof mascara. If you can, it is better not to use any mascara at all. You may find youdon't even need it! If you must make sure it is water based.
- Avoid running water over your face for long periods of time. Moisture will break down the bond of the glue.
- Avoid rubbing your eyes or lashes, especially when washing your face. Use your fingertips to gently cleanse the eyes and then splash water on your face.
- Avoid using an eyelash curler. One of the benefits of lash extensions is the ability to add curl toyour lashes. If you would like more curl, please speak to your technician.
- If you can, sleep on your back to avoid the risk of lashes rubbing against your pillow.
- Gently brush your lashes with a mascara wand to groom them. The best time to do this is aftershowering, as they will be softer and less likely to damage.
- Avoid pulling your lashes, and do not attempt to remove them yourself. If you would like themremoved, please contact your technician.

If you experience any pain, redness or irritation, contact your technician immediately.

Eyelash Extension Aftercare

- Do not tint your natural eyelashes immediately after lash extension application. Tint may be done before the application begins and/or at fills before the application begins.
- Do not use a regular eyelash curler that crimps the eyelashes. Heated wand curlers may be used.
- Do not rub your eyes or lashes when washing your face. Clean around the eyes with your fingertips and then gently splash water on your face.
- Do not pull your lash extensions, as it will take out your own natural eyelash as well.
- Do not go in a sauna while wearing eyelash extensions for extended periods of time.
- Do not use mascara. If you must only use mascara especially formulated for

Aftercare Card

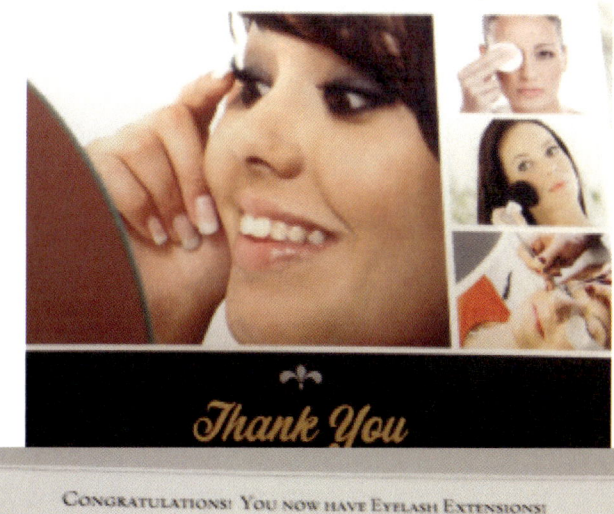

I like to use Vistaprint.com for my marketing materials. You have to spell check yourself.

You'll notice in the second "do's" it says hated eyelash curlers instead of heated eyelash curlers.

Triple check that spelling when using services like these!!

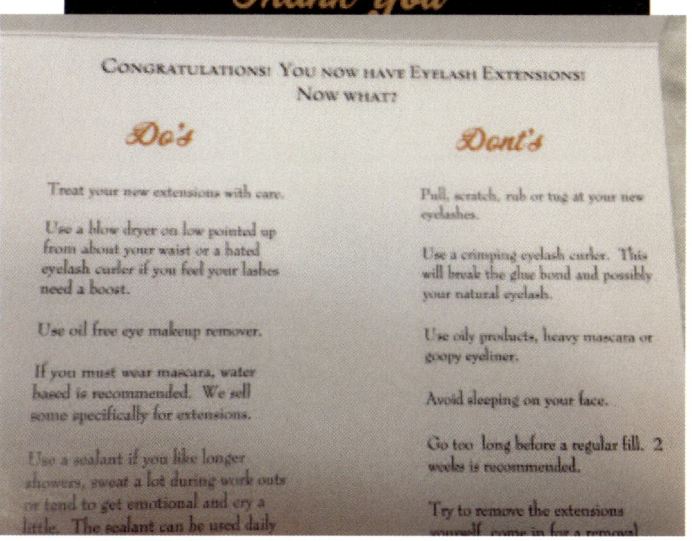

Eyelash Extension Menu

Full Set
$250

Standard 2 week fill	$55
Diva 1 week fill	40
Re-Fringe	75-180

If you come in with less than 10 extensions per eye a re-fringe is necessary, you will be charged according to amount of work needed

Mink Full Set
$350

Standard 2 week mink fill	$85
Diva 1 week mink fill	65
Re-Fringe mink	125-290
Removal	$30-50

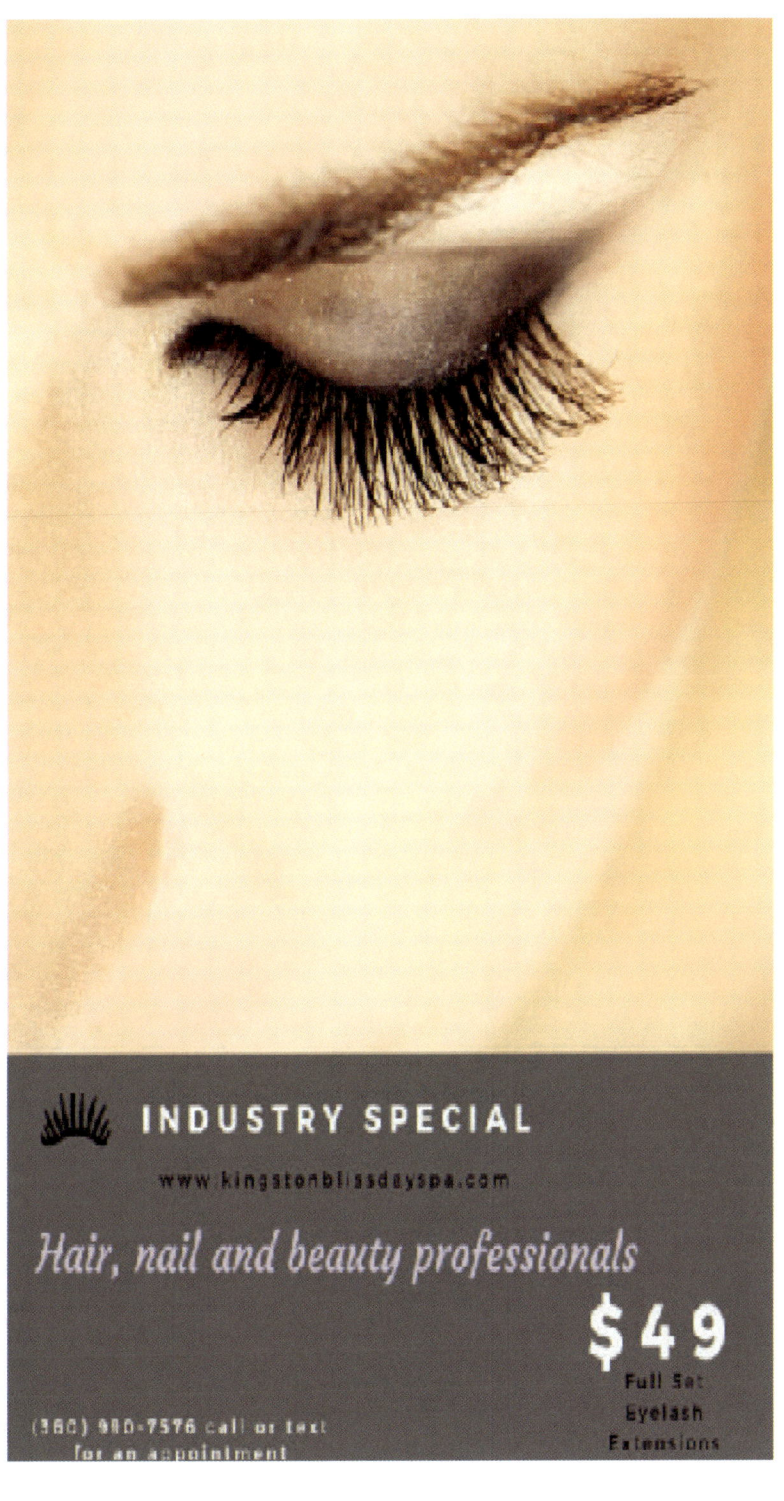

An industry special is for other beauty professionals. Getting extensions on hair stylists, nail techs and other public figures is a great way to have walking advertisements. Setting a super low price will entice them to come in, yet still value your time and product expenses.

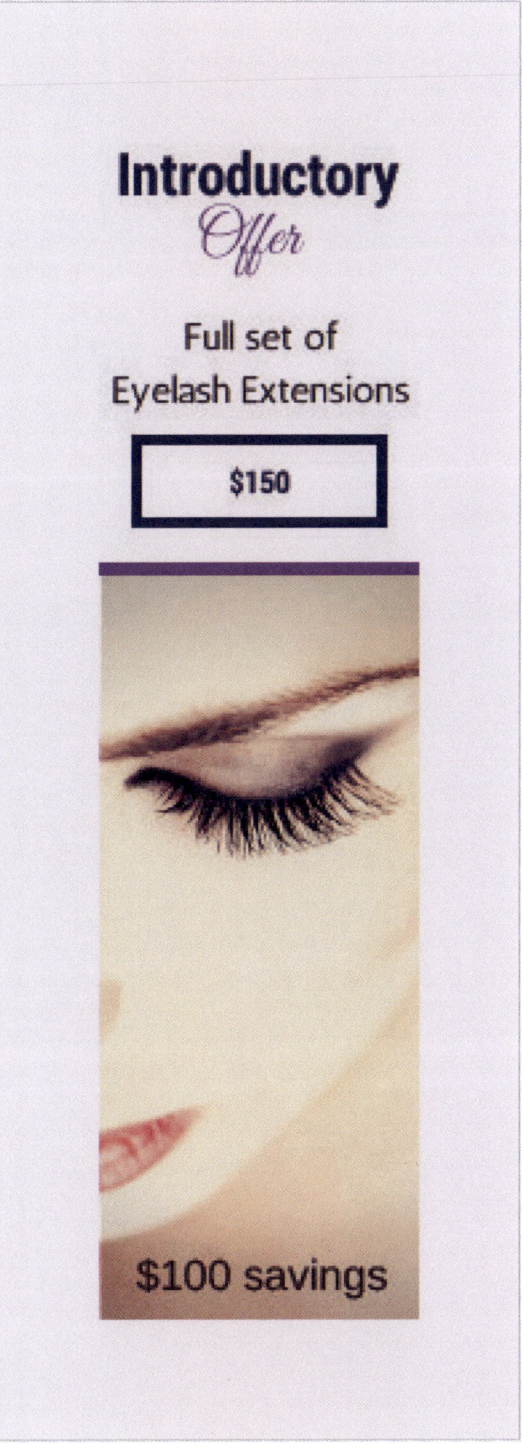

Printed in Great Britain
by Amazon